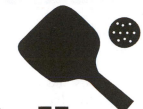

Pickle-Ball
For Player and Teacher
3rd Edition

Joyce M. Curtis, P.E.D.
Abilene Christian University

Morton Publishing Company
925 West Kenyon, Unit 12
Englewood, Colorado 80110

⊜ ACKNOWLEDGMENTS

For aid in the preparation of this book, I want to thank Julie Larson and Cassandra Weyandt, who did the photography. Sincere thanks go to Andrea Hunt and Donna Stone, Abilene Christian University students who were subjects for the pictures. I am grateful to Jean Shafer for typing the first drafts of the material for class, to Jill Massie for typing and retyping the manuscript many times, and to Beth McLeskey for her comments and suggestions on the manuscript.

I also want to thank the many new Pickle-Ball players at Abilene Christian University who are excited about the game and gave much encouragement in the development of this material.

A special thanks is extended to Mr. Doug Smith, general manager of Pickle-Ball, Inc., for his encouragement and help in collecting materials about the development of the game and for supplying information and pictures to keep up-to-date in Pickle-Ball happenings for this third edition.

Also for the third edition, I appreciate the time given by Abilene Christian Exercise Science and Health majors Kade Burns, Moses Hall, Blake Lindsey, and Brooke Stephens for being subjects for the action pictures.

I appreciate the assistance of Dickie Hill, Ph.D., Professor of Exercise Science an Health, Abilene Christian University, in developing the new Chapter 2, "Fitness and Athletic Performance."

Also, many thanks to Bob Curtis of Curtis Photography for taking the new action pictures for this third edition.

Printed in the United States of America

ISBN: 0-89582-459-0

⊕ FOREWORD

The original purpose of Pickle-Ball was to provide a game that the whole family might enjoy regardless of athletic ability or strength. In 1965, our family would have never dreamed that someday more than 200,000 people would be playing Pickle-Ball in school physical education programs, YMCAs, parks and recreation centers, and camps, and on private courts in backyards and driveways. Pickle-Ball has enjoyed widespread growth throughout the United States and Canada. The Pickle-Ball movement has been growing among senior adults in Singapore and Japan. The main growth of Pickle-Ball, however, continues to be in elementary, middle school, high school, and college physical education programs. Most physical education professionals find Pickle-Ball to be the ideal game to teach racquet skills, and it is an excellent lead-up game for teaching tennis. Thousand of physical education professionals have incorporated a Pickle-Ball unit into their physical education curriculum.

Pickle-Ball continues to receive widespread support among physical education professionals at all grade levels and is being actively introduced by recreation directors at camps. YMCAs, parks and recreation centers, and athletic clubs. Pickle-Ball, Inc. continues to manufacture and distribute high-quality wood paddles, balls, nets, and sets, which are purchased directly from schools and institutions or through team sporting goods stores and institutional physical education supply catalogs.

The growth in Pickle-Ball has not been limited to institutional settings. Many families have purchased the new portable Tournament sets and set them up in driveways and cul-de-sacs. Further, families have installed asphalt/concrete multipurpose game courts in their backyards so they can play Pickle-Ball. Many retirement communities are building courts as part of their planned exercise and recreational program. Pickle-Ball promotes exercise, friendship, and aerobic fitness.

I would like to extend our thanks and appreciation to Dr. Curtis for her tremendous efforts in compiling the first in-depth presentation of the game of Pickle-Ball in a fashion that will greatly assist physical education professionals.

Douglas Smith, President, Pickle-Ball, Inc.
801 N.W. 48th St., Seattle, WA 98107
207-784-4723   FAX 206-781-0782

⬭ PREFACE

This book brings together a body of knowledge for present and future Pickle-Ball enthusiasts. Information is presented concerning the origin and development of the game, the basic skills, the rules as they have evolved to the present time, and the tactics and strategy to help the player develop his own pattern of play to the best of his ability.

The new Chapter 2, Fitness and Athletic Performance, should help the Pickle-Ball player to develop the physical components needed to become a successful player. The chapter contains specific physical performance activities to be incorporated into the individual development plan.

The Chapter 3, on basic Pickle-Ball skills, should be helpful to the beginning player. It describes common errors and gives suggestions on how to correct them.

The Chapter 8, on game strategy used in singles and doubles, should be particularly helpful to students and teachers alike.

The Chapter 9, a collection of practice drills, will be helpful to teachers in preparing class progressions and activities.

The chapter on evaluation, (Chapter 10) presents Pickle-Ball skills tests and references for other tests.

Appendix 2 provides sample lesson plans for Pickle-Ball classes.

⬡ TABLE OF CONTENTS

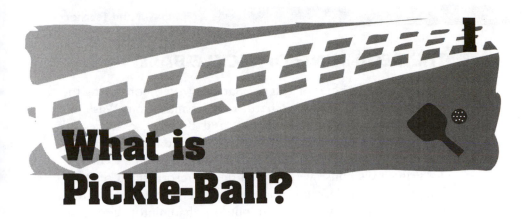

What is Pickle-Ball?

The key to the rapidly increasing popularity of Pickle-Ball® is that it is easy to learn and is enjoyed across the spectrum of men, women, and children. The first time you play, you will attain confidence, regardless of your level of athletic ability. At the same time, the competitive individual will find this sport demanding and challenging enough to make him or her want to play regularly.

Winning Pickle-Ball will be the result of putting the ball where you want, controlling the tempo of the game, and keeping the ball in play. Size and strength are not major factors in who will win the game. Strategy and tactics tend to be just as important to the final outcome.

Pickle-Ball is an ideal family sport. Mixed doubles are great fun, with father and daughter trying their skill against mother and son. In singles, father versus daughter and mother versus son games provide outstanding family entertainment and fitness.

The small court size allows for long rallies and a variety of play by players determined to win over their opponent. The fast volley exchanges increase the fun for players and spectators alike. Pickle-Ball is played by two or four people on a court identical in size to a badminton doubles court. Easily lowering the net to 3 feet on the badminton doubles court will convert it to a Pickle-Ball court. Lightweight paddles (slightly larger than Ping-Pong paddles) and the plastic perforated ball are the keys to producing long, exciting rallies consisting of volleys at the net and ground strokes similar to tennis. Pickle-Ball strategies include the lob, overhead, smash, passing shots by the opponent at the net, and fast volley exchanges.

®Pickle-Ball is the registered trademark of Pickle-Ball, Incorporated of Seattle, Washington.

THE BEGINNING OF PICKLE-BALL

After playing 18 holes of golf one Saturday afternoon during the summer of 1965, Joel Pritchard, congressman from Washington's First Congressional District, and Bill Bell, a successful businessman, returned to Pritchard's home and found their families sitting around complaining that "there's nothing to do."

Pritchard's house was located on the resort island of Bainbridge — a short ferryboat ride west from Seattle, Washington. On the property was an old outdoor badminton court, so Pritchard and Bell decided that badminton would be the activity for the afternoon and began trying to find some usable equipment. They could not find a full set of playable badminton equipment, so they began to improvise with what was available. They cut off the shafts of the damaged rackets, found a perforated plastic ball, and began to play.

The players had trouble hitting the plastic ball, which was about 3 inches in diameter, with the short-handled, small-headed rackets. The determined fathers soon came up with four solid wooden paddles that are similar to the official paddles of today.

At first they placed the badminton net at regulation height of 5 feet, and the players volleyed the balls back and forth over the net with pleasure and excitement. Everyone liked the feeling of the plastic ball rebounding from the wooden paddles. The holes in the ball slowed it down, and the flight was much like the flight of a feathered shuttlecock.

The players soon realized that the ball would bounce well and true from the solid asphalt surface of the court. By allowing the ball to bounce, a new dimension was added to the new game they were creating.

The next morning, when Pritchard and Bell came down for breakfast, they discovered that the others were already outside playing their new game. The net had been lowered to approximately the height of a tennis net, and the women and children were making hard drives and volleying the ball at the net.

The rest of the day was spent just having fun and batting the ball back and forth over the net. The players had no scoring system and no formal rules. No one was competitive in the play. Pritchard and Bell had discovered something that everyone likes to do.

The next weekend Barney McCallum came out for a visit, was introduced to the new game, and got hooked on it.

Pritchard, Bell, and McCallum enjoyed hitting the ball over the net but became bored with doing only that. So they began to draw up some playing rules to make the game more competitive.

The original purpose was for the whole family to play together, so this was a prime consideration in formulating rules. They drew up the rules easily, depending heavily on badminton. In their first version, only the serving team could score points; servers had to make their deliveries underhand (so the serve was easy and did not become an overpowering offensive weapon), and the service was alternated so one opposing player and then the other received it.

The server was allowed to step over the baseline with one foot so a tree in one corner of the court would not obstruct the delivery. (Only one foot had to remain behind the baseline before the ball was hit.) As in badminton, only one serve was allowed, and the paddle had to meet the ball below the server's waist.

The competitive players soon discovered that the best position was right on top of the net. From here, it was simple to put away the ball with a volley or smash. The men decided they needed some control at the net, so they created the "penalty zone" between the short service line of the badminton court and the net and a player standing within it could not volley. Only after a short shot had bounced in that area of the court could a player enter the "penalty area" to make a return. This new rule controlled the net player's advantage and contributed to the making of the game. Later the line was moved back to 7 feet from the net, and the area was renamed the "non-volley zone."

The Pritchards' cocker spaniel, named Pickles, became interested in the new game. He would lie and watch the game from a distance and a loose ball would come his way, he would take it and disappear. Thus, the name "Pickle-Ball" was born.

THE EVOLUTION OF PICKLE-BALL

During the following winter, Barney McCallum kept wanting to play the new game. One day while looking out his window, he realized that the street in front of his house was about the width of a Pickle-Ball court. A few minutes later he determined that the street was 22 feet wide. He and his son Dave lined off a court and set up net posts that could be tipped over, as cars occasionally drove on his dead-end street.

Not long after, McCallum added another innovation to the game: the double-bounce rule. This rule stated that the opposing team could hit its first shot only after the ball had first bounced on the playing surface. The receiving team had to let the ball bounce, and the serving team had to let the return of serve bounce. Only after these two bounces could the ball be volleyed in a rally. This diminished the advantage of the serving team and gave some edge to the receiving team, as the receiver could take the net with a deep approach shot on receiving serve. (The non-volley zone still controlled the net player's strength.)

During the winter of 1967, the first permanent Pickle-Ball court in the United States was constructed in Joel Pritchard's backyard in Seattle, Washington. Soon, another followed at a neighbor's house across the street from Barney McCallum's house. From 1965 to 1973, the founding fathers and friends played the game faithfully. Fewer than 10 courts were established during the 8-year span.

On October 8, 1997, Joel Pritchard died at age 72. Mr. Pritchard had given 32 years of public service as a state legislator, congressman and lieutenant governor. He never was well known in Washington politics and was better known for his connection to the game of Pickle-Ball.

The most effective advertising for this new game was word of mouth. Most people really liked the game and told their friends about it. Some of the local high schools and colleges added it to their physical education classes. They already had badminton courts, and Pickle-Ball could be easily added.

In 1972, a corporation was formed to protect the new creation, although the three original stockholders did not expect to give their full time to the business. The corporation published the playing rules and copyrighted them. "Pickle-Ball" became the registered trademark of Pickle-Ball Inc. Seattle, WA.

By the mid-1970s, Pickle-Ball had spread into almost all the high schools and junior colleges in the greater Western Washington area. The Seattle Parks and Recreation Department began promoting the game to seniors. The community centers were empty during the day, so the parks department promoted Pickle-Ball for senior adults to increase the use of their facilities and to promote health, fitness, and exercise for senior adults.

In June of 1975, *The National Observer* carried an article about Pickle-Ball, and in 1976, *Tennis* magazine did an article on "America's newest racquet sport." This national publicity brought inquiries from all parts of the United States and orders for paddles, balls, and playing instructions.[1]

By 1990, Pickle-Ball was being played in all 50 states. The United States of America Pickle-Ball Association organized 10 to 15 tournaments in the Puget Sound area. Several hundred older Seattle-area residents play Pickle-Ball at some 15 Seattle-area senior centers, parks and recreation departments, and community centers. Leesburg, Florida has Pickle-Ball leagues, and competition begins at 10 a.m. once a week. In the past few years, one center has built 12 courts for Pickle-Ball, and more are on the drawing board. Another center has completed four Pickle-Ball courts.

Pickle-Ball is played in many church recreation programs throughout the United States. Many church directors consider Pickle-Ball a great addition for their youth programs and senior adult health and fitness programs.

Pickle-Ball is presently being introduced at state physical education conventions and advertised in recreation and physical education journals. Most school supply catalogs include Pickle-Ball equipment.

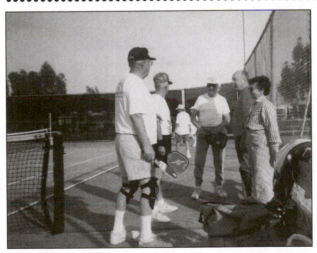

Senior citizens waiting to play at Desert Springs, California.

PHOTO COURTESY OF WARREN COCHRANE, SEATTLE, WA

FIGURE 1.1

---

[1] Dick Squires, *The Other Racquet Sports* (McGraw-Hill, 1978), pp. 228–232.

Review Questions

Completion

1. Winning Pickle-Ball will be the result of putting the ball _____

   _____, controlling the _____,

   and keeping _____.

2. The Pickle-Ball court is identical to a _____
   in size.

3. The game of Pickle-Ball was created in the summer of _____

   in the state of _____.

4. In developing the game, the server was allowed to step over the base-

   line so that _____.

5. Where did the name Pickle-Ball come from? _____

   _____.

6. The serve was made with an underhand motion so it did not become

   _____.

7. The purpose of the non-volley zone is to control the _____

   _____.

8. The _____ was created
   to govern and promote the game of Pickle-Ball.

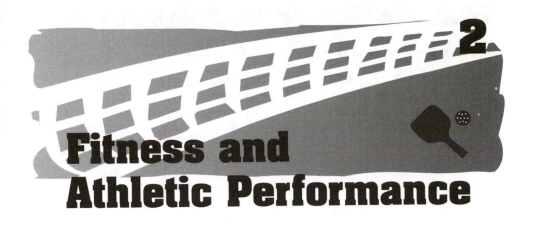

Fitness and Athletic Performance

Many factors contribute to success in a sport. A good baseball player needs strength to throw and hit a ball, speed to run the bases, hand-eye coordination to catch, agility to scramble for a hard-hit ground ball, and endurance to last a twilight double-header. A gymnast needs upper-body strength to hold a position on the rings, agility and balance for the balance beam, and precise body control for a perfect dismount. A cyclist needs cardiovascular capacity to ride for hours, as well as quadriceps strength and endurance to pedal up long hills. A soccer player needs strength to kick, cardiovascular capacity to run for 90 minutes, leg speed for quick bursts, and skill for ball control.

ELEMENTS OF FITNESS

Figure 2.1 depicts the components that contribute to performance. At the base are those that lay the foundation. The next two layers consist of physical variables. Then the emotional/psychological factors come into play. In actual performance, the two most significant factors are skill and mental attitude.

Each component of fitness is independent. A person can develop endurance without speed or strength without agility. Some athletes are highly fit in one area and under average in another. Fitness also is sport-specific. For example, an athlete may be able to run a sub-4-minute mile but unable to swim a length of the neighborhood pool. A swimmer may knock off a 15-minute mile in the pool but take twice the world-class running time on the track. Through years of practice in the water, a person will need to develop the swimming muscles of his or her upper body, learn proper stroking techniques, gain a feel for the water, and acquire all the other skills necessary for

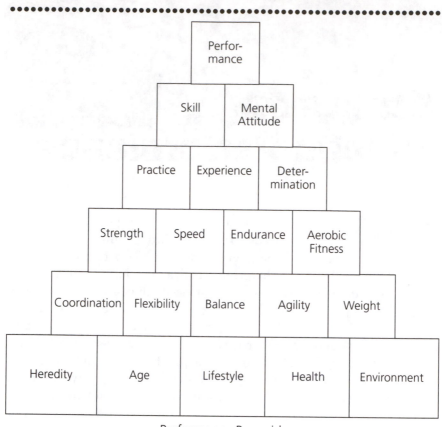

Performance Pyramid.

FIGURE 2.1 ●●●

excellence in swimming. No activity will improve performance at a given sport better than sport-specific practice.

Fitness does not guarantee athletic performance. The winner of the Olympic decathlon is considered to be the world's best athlete for that year. Many other athletes, however, can achieve better results in the individual decathlon events.

Selective fitness training can improve performance. All athletes use their unique abilities to enhance their performance. Intelligent athletes take stock of their abilities and strengthen the weaknesses while refining the strengths. Readers might think about what is required for the sport in which they are interested and how they measure up.[1]

---

[1] *Sports Fitness and Training,* by Richard Mangie, Peter Jaki, and O. William Dayton (New York: Pantheon Books, 1987, pp. 11–14).

Everyone can enjoy Pickle-Ball. The long rallies aid in developing cardiovascular fitness. The stretching and twisting develop flexibility. The game promotes agility and coordination. It requires fast reflexes, good physical conditioning, and concentration. It is also a social game and makes an excellent family recreation activity.[2]

Pickle-Ball consumes a lot of energy in a short time, making it an ideal form of workout for people on tight schedules. The length of the rallies between skilled, evenly matched opponents requires a heavy expenditure of calories. With the exception of a few minor aches and pains generally associated with strenuous physical activity, a Pickle-Ball player rarely is injured. The ultralightweight equipment precludes even tennis elbow and tendonitis. The skills and techniques used in Pickle-Ball can be carried over effectively to other activities, such as racquetball, tennis, badminton, paddleball, and squash.[3]

This chapter covers the components of physical fitness: flexibility, cardiovascular endurance, muscular endurance, muscular strength, and body composition. Exercise specific to each of these components are included.

FLEXIBILITY

Flexibility is the range of motion in a joint. It is the ability to bend without "breaking"; not stiff or rigid; easily bent. Dynamic flexibility is a nonrestrictive range of normal joint motion as a result of muscular contraction. Static flexibility is the extended range of motion available to a body joint without injury. Exercise sessions normally begin and end with flexibility and stretching exercises. Thus, it is an adjunct to cardiovascular exercise and strength training. It is a necessary component of all forms of exercise, to prevent injuries and maximize the workout.

Flexibility is developed through regular effort and can diminish when efforts cease. Flexibility also delays the aging process.

In sum, good flexibility:

1. Decreases susceptibility to injury.

2. Reduces susceptibility to chronic lower back pain.

3. Increases physical performance in certain activities.

---

[2] *Badminton Today*, by Tariq Wadood (St. Paul: West Publishing, 1990), p. 2.

[3] *Badminton*, by Jack Reznik and Ron Byrd (Scottsdale, AZ: Gorsuch Scarisbrick, 1987), pp. 3–4.

4. Is essential for total fitness.

5. Delays some effects of aging.

Poor flexibility can be a result of anatomical limitations, and weak muscles. A sedentary lifestyle is a major cause.

Some criteria for flexibility exercises are that:

1. Each joint must be stretched for full benefit.

2. The session must include warm up and warm down.

3. Sustained positions that gradually and gently extend the muscles are most effective (20–60 seconds).

4. Maximum stretches are needed and these must be painless. Dynamic types of stretching (bouncing) should be avoided, as they can cause injuries.

5. Flexibility exercises should be combined with strength training and aerobic training.

6. Flexibility exercises should be done three or four times a week. Even once a week is better than none. Reducing excess body fat will make optimum flexibility more attainable.

A person's level of flexibility is normally measured through the following:

1. Sit and reach: hips, lower back

2. Shoulder hyperextension: shoulders

3. Trunk hyperextension: back

Value of Flexibility for Pickle-Ball

Pickle-Ball is a fast-paced sport, requiring jumping and lunging. Poor flexibility carries the risk of strained muscles. Good flexibility can help in reducing delayed muscle soreness following strenuous tournaments.[4] It allows you to move smoothly through a full range of motion in every stroke and serve.[5]

Specifically:

1. Players must reach for the ball.

2. Players must bend the body to hit round-the-head strokes.

3. Players must be able to reach and stretch to their body's limits without being injured.[6]

---

[4] *Badminton,* 4th edition (Prospect Heights, IL: Waveland Press, 1996), p. 133.

[5] *Badminton Today,* p. 108.

[6] *Teaching Badminton,* by Ralph B. Ballou (Minneapolis: Burgess Publishing, 1982), p. 134.

4. Flexibility is critical to the prevention of injuries.

5. It is desirable to stretch the shoulders and inner thigh muscles, because they undergo the greatest strain during play and are most subject to injury.[7]

Specific Stretches for Pickle-Ball Players

EXERCISE •••••••••••••••••••••••••••••••••••• Plantar Arch

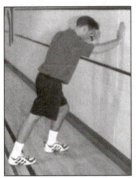

1. Stand upright 2 or 3 steps from a wall.
2. Bend one leg forward and keep the opposite leg straight.

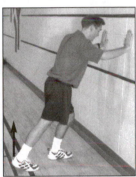

3. Lean slightly against the wall.
4. Keep your rear foot down, flat, and parallel to your hips.
5. Exhale, raise the rear heel off the floor, shifting your weight onto the ball of your rear foot, and press downward.
6. Hold the stretch and relax.

EXERCISE •••••••••••••••••••••••••• Ankles/Anterior Lower Leg

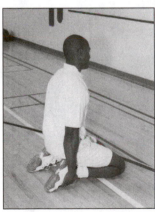

1. Kneel on all fours with your toes pointing backward. If this is uncomfortable, place a blanket under your shins.
2. Exhale, and slowly sit on your heels (if you can).
3. Reach around, grasp the top portion of your toes, and pull them toward your head.
4. Hold the stretch and relax.

(This stretch is used to prevent shin-splints.)

(Do not use with bad knees.)

---

[7] *Badminton: Basic Skills and Drills,* by Roger L. Sweeting and Janet S. Wilson (Mountain View, CA: Mayfield, 1992), p. 74.

EXERCISE •••••••••••••••••••••••••••••••••• **Achilles Tendon**

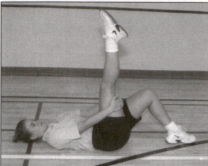

1. Lie on your back with legs extended.
2. Flex one leg and slide the foot toward the buttocks.
3. Raise the opposite leg toward your face and grasp behind the knee.
4. Exhale, and slowly flex the foot toward your face.
5. Hold the stretch and relax.

If you have a bad back, flex the extended leg and slowly lower it to the floor.

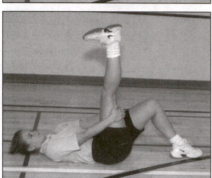

EXERCISE •••••••••••••••••••••••••••••••••• **Achilles Tendon**

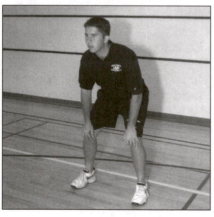 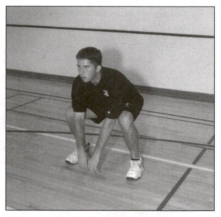

1. Stand upright with both hands on your hips or knees. If necessary, hold onto a wall for balance.
2. Keep your heels down, flat, and parallel.
3. Exhale, and slowly flex your knees, bringing them as close to the floor as possible.
4. Hold the stretch and relax.

EXERCISE •• **Hamstrings**

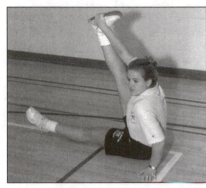

1. Sit upright on the floor, hands behind your hips for support and your legs extended.
2. Flex one knee and grasp the instep of your foot with one hand.
3. Exhale, and slowly extend your leg until it reaches a 90-degree angle.
4. Hold the stretch and relax.

EXERCISE •• **Adductors**

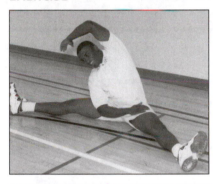

1. Sit upright on the floor with both legs straight.
2. Straddle your legs as wide as possible.
3. Drop one arm and raise your other arm overhead.
4. Exhale, rotate your trunk, and extend your upper torso onto your leg.
5. Hold the stretch and relax.

EXERCISE •• **Quadriceps**

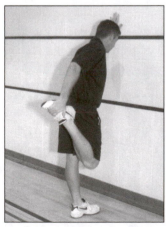

1. Stand upright with one hand against a surface for balance and support.
2. Flex one leg and raise the foot to your buttocks.
3. Slightly flex the supporting leg.
4. Exhale, reach down, grasp your raised foot with one hand, and pull your heel toward your buttocks without overcompressing the knee.
5. Hold the stretch and relax.

(Do not use with bad knees.)

EXERCISE ••••••••••••••••••••••••••••••••••• **Buttocks and Hips**

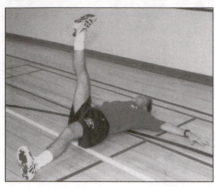 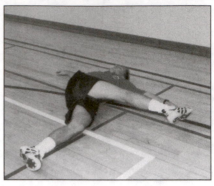

1. Lie flat on your back with one leg raised and straight and your arms out to your sides.
2. Exhale, and slowly lower your raised leg to the opposite hand while keeping your elbows, head, and shoulders flat on the floor.
3. Hold the stretch and relax.

••

EXERCISE •••••••••••••••••••••••••••••••••• **Lateral Trunk**

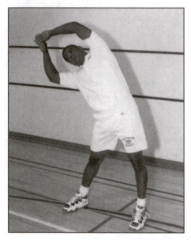

1. Stand upright with feet slightly apart and hands interlocking overhead.
2. Exhale, drop one ear toward your shoulder, and slowly lower your arms sideways.
3. Hold the stretch and relax.

••

EXERCISE•••••••••••••••••••••••••••••••••• **Anterior Shoulder**

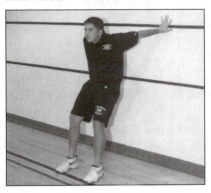

1. Stand upright, with your hands behind your hips at about shoulder height, resting on a wall, and your fingers pointing upward.
2. Exhale, and flex your legs to lower your shoulders.
3. Hold the stretch and relax.

EXERCISE •••••••••••••••••••••••••••••••• **Internal Rotators**

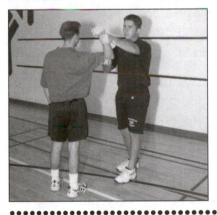

1. Stand upright with your right arm raised to shoulder height and flexed to a right angle.
2. Your partner stands in front of you and to your side, grasping your right wrist with his or her left hand and supporting your right elbow with his or her right hand.
3. Exhale as you allow your partner to gently push your wrist backward and downward. Communicate with your partner and use great care.
4. Hold the stretch and relax.

EXERCISE ••••••••••••••••••••••••••••••••• **Wrist Extensors**

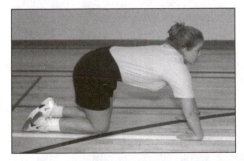

1. Kneel on the floor, flex your wrists, and place the tops of your hands on the floor.
2. Exhale, and lean against the floor.
3. Hold the stretch and relax.

⊕ CARDIOVASCULAR (CV) ENDURANCE

Cardio refers to the heart, and vascular refers to the system of vessels for conveying blood. Thus, cardiovascular (CV) function is the capacity of the heart, lungs, and blood vessels to fuel increased physical activity. Cardiovascular fitness is the ability of the heart, blood vessels, blood, and respiratory system to supply fuel, especially oxygen, to the muscles and the ability of the muscles to utilize fuel to allow sustained exercise.

Cardiovascular fitness improves one's physiological functioning by:

1. slowing the resting heart rate.
2. increasing cardiac output or blood volume pumped from the heart.
3. increasing the elasticity of blood vessels.
4. often lowering resting blood pressure.
5. improving oxygen carrying capacity.
6. improving coronary circulation.

Cardiovascular exercise delays the degenerative effects of aging and some evidence shows improved resistance to disease in general. Psychological factors often related to stress can be improved by raising the self-esteem, elevating one's status among peers, decreasing depression and anxiety, reducing muscular tension, and increasing endorphins, allowing the body to better withstand stress.

Some reasons for poor CV endurance are laziness, procrastination, physical limitations, and the person thinks he or she is "too busy." Development of cardiovascular fitness requires a person to follow certain criteria while exercising, as follows. The *exercise mode* must use the large muscles and has to be rhythmical in nature. The *intensity* must be 60%–90% of estimated maximum heart rate. The formulas are:

$$\text{minimum} = (220 - \text{age}) \times .60$$
$$\text{maximum} = (220 - \text{age}) \times .90$$

The *duration* of the activity must be continuous for 20–60 minutes. Less intensity requires longer duration, and higher intensity requires shorter duration. The *frequency* of exercise must be three to five times a week. Three is considered minimum and should help maintain a current level of fitness. Four is moderate and should improve fitness. Five or six days is a heavy exercise schedule and will create more rapid improvement. Exercising all seven days a week is overdoing it and is not recommended for general fitness.

CV endurance can be measured by the following assessments.

1. *Submaximal test.* This may consist of a one-mile walk (clocking the time) or a 12-minute jog or walk. Other methods, such as step tests and stair climbing also are used.

2. *Treadmill test.* Maximal physical effort is required to determine CV fitness. After total or near total exertion for 20 minutes or more the pulse is checked 5 minutes into the recovery time. It should be lower than 120 beats per minute. The lower the rate, the better.

In sum, in cardiovascular endurance exercise, the activity must be aerobic in nature. The person must participate at least three times a week, in a mode, intensity, duration, and frequency to maintain or increase fitness.

Value of CV Endurance for Pickle-Ball

Pickle-Ball is an explosive game played discontinuously. This means that *anaerobic* power dominates.* To more effectively deliver the oxygen to the muscles during the recovery intervals between rallies, some degree of *aerobic* fitness is called for. The key is to develop *anaerobic* and *aerobic* fitness simultaneously in a pattern specific to the demands of Pickle-Ball.[8]

Specific Exercises for Pickle-Ball

Specific exercises that will aid participants in Pickle-Ball include the following:

1. *Short sprints* at maximum to near maximum speed, separated by quick stops and intervals of walking.

2. *Distance running* (aerobic): Less sufficient but does improve stamina.[9]

---

*Muscular activity of a short duration that requires little or no oxygen during contractions, so the energy level is replenished between periods of activity.

[8] *Badminton*, pp. 91–92.

[9] *Badminton*.

3. *Shadow drills:* The player, at medium and then full speed, simulates playing a game by moving about the court making simulated replies to the shots of an imaginary opponent.[10]

4. *Line touching drills* (anaerobic): Involve changes of direction.

5. *Aerobic activities:* Increase the endurance necessary for long matches.

6. *Anaerobic* activities: Help condition the heart and lungs for the quick bursts of energy typically needed during long rallies.[11]

MUSCULAR ENDURANCE

Muscular endurance relates to fatigability of the skeletal muscles. *Dynamic muscular endurance* is the ability to exert continuous force or perform repetitions against submaximal resistance in a given time. It is also called *isotonic endurance.* *Static muscular endurance* refers to a muscle's ability to remain contracted for a long period. This is usually measured by the length of time a person can hold a body position and is called *isometric endurance.*

Muscular endurance enables a person to perform daily vocational activities and be able to participate in various recreational activities after a day of work. It increases static strength of bones, ligaments, and tendons, as well as lean body mass. It improves the blood lipid (fat) profile and thereby reduces the risk for cardiovascular disease. The improved physical appearance can enhance the self-concept as well.

The muscles will degenerate if a person does not engage in proper activities. The phrase "use it or lose it" applies here. Possible reasons for muscular decline include the following.

1. Being a "couch potato" — simply not exercising;

2. An extended illness or injury that prevent exercising;

3. Not being consistent with one's exercise program.

4. Personal physiological limitations.

5. Not exercising at a level considered to be aerobic in nature.

---

[10] *Badminton for Beginners,* by Ralph Balow (Englewood, CO: Morton, 1992), p. 65.
[11] *Badminton: Basic Skills and Drills,* p. 75.

Muscular endurance can be developed through the following guidelines for a given exercise.

1. *Resistance:* Should be light to medium, usually no more than 50% of maximum capacity;

2. *Repetitions:* Muscle should become fatigued, but only after a minimum of 20 repetitions;

3. *Duration:* Can be continued for multiple sets or for an extended period; at least two or three times per week.

Measuring muscular endurance for single muscles is not practical or necessary. Specific groups of muscles are of more importance. Examples are the back, abdominal muscles, upper arms and shoulders, lower arms, and lower legs. The following tests are used to measure muscular endurance.

1. Total number of push-ups (dynamic for shoulders and upper arms)

2. Number of sit-ups performed in 2 minutes (dynamic for abdominals)

3. Sitting tucks (dynamic) for total number (dynamic for abdominals)

4. 90-degree push-up (dynamic for shoulders, chest, and upper arms)

5. Flexed-arm support for time (static for shoulders, chest, and upper arms)

6. Stationary leg change (dynamic for legs and hips)

7. Half-squats (dynamic for thighs and buttocks)

Muscular endurance can be maintained by following the same procedures as for muscular development. One exception could be fewer days per week. If the muscles are not exercised, muscular endurance will be lost. Three times per week for the endurance activity should maintain the current level. A desire for increased endurance would require an increase in the duration of the activity or an increase in the number of exercise sessions per week.

Value of Muscular Endurance for Pickle-Ball

If your legs tire after an hour of Pickle-Ball, or your basic shots are no longer effective after an hour of Pickle-Ball, you are probably experiencing muscle fatigue associated with poor endurance. Also, late in the afternoon of a tournament, if you cannot run as quickly as you did early in the morning, you are probably experiencing muscle fatigue.

Specific Exercises for Pickle-Ball

Long rallies in Pickle-Ball demand both cardiorespiratory and muscular endurance. The running required in Pickle-Ball demands that the muscles of the legs have a fair endurance capacity. To attain muscular endurance for Pickle-Ball, participants should use as many game-like drills as possible. This is to include work on explosive movements to all four corners of the court, drills to increase foot speed, reactions, and ability to move quickly around the court for a designated time.

⊕ MUSCULAR STRENGTH

Absolute strength is defined as one's ability to exert force against a resistance, usually maximal. *Relative strength* is the amount of force one can exert in relation to one's body weight or per unit of muscle cross-section.

Muscular strength allows a person to perform daily vocational activities and still have enough strength to participate in various recreational activities. Strength training is also used to rehabilitate an injured body muscle or muscles. A side benefit of strength training is the confidence gained from the improved physical appearance.

A major benefit of muscular strength is that it reduces the risk for injury. Also, additional calories can be expended because of the increased muscle mass. Muscular strength helps to develop the body's vascular or circulatory system. Finally, strength training increases bone mass and thus decreases the onset or severity of osteoporosis.

The axiom "use it or lose it" can be applied to muscular strength. No matter how much muscular strength a person has, it will decline if the level of activity decreases. A person's muscular strength might be low or decline for the following reasons:

1. Being "couch potato" — simply not exercising.

2. An extended illness or injury which would prevent exercising.

3. Not exercising consistently.

4. Personal physical limitations.

5. Not exercising at a level sufficient to maintain the current level.

6. Working certain muscles while neglecting others.

Muscular strength can be developed by following guidelines for a given exercise.

1. *Resistance:* Should be classified as heavy (usually at least 60% to 80% of one's maximum capacity.)
2. *Repetitions:* Should fatigue a muscle within a few (5–10) repetitions.
3. *Duration:* Should continue for additional sets of repetitions following a brief (less than 5 minutes) rest interval and should be done at least two or three times per week.

The strength of individual muscles can be measured, as can groups of muscles. An individual's personal goals and objectives influence the measurement process. To determine if muscular strength is being maintained or improving, evaluation should be conducted from time to time. The following methods can be used for measuring muscular strength.

1. Hand dynamometer: to measure grip strength (isometric)
2. Pull-ups: To measure arm and shoulder strength.
3. Trunk lift: To measure upper back and neck muscles.
4. Squat lifting: For legs and lower back.
5. Free-weights: To evaluate all muscles.

Muscular strength will decline if the muscles are not regularly challenged. Muscular strength can be maintained by following the same procedures as in muscle development. One exception could be that one may be able to exercise fewer days per week. Two or three times per week should maintain a current level. If increased strength is desired, additional resistance is required.

Value of Muscular Strength for Pickle-Ball

In Pickle-Ball, muscular strength enables the participant to hit the ball harder and to continue doing this for the duration of a long match.[12] Also, strong muscles are less susceptible to injury.

Specific Exercises for Pickle-Ball

Quadriceps and calf strength is needed to move quickly to every shot. Abdominal, forearm, and shoulder strength are essential

---

[12] *Badminton, 4th edition,* p. 133.

to hit through the ball quickly and effortlessly. Wrist strength is necessary for every shot.[13] Therefore, strength training should target these muscle groups.

BODY COMPOSITION

Body composition is the ratio of fat to non-fat (lean) tissue. Another way to define body composition is the relative percentage of muscle, fat, bone, and other tissues of which the body is composed. A fit person has a relatively low (but not too low) percentage of body fat. *Obesity* is a condition in which a person's percent of body fat reaches a level of 20% for men and 30% for women. Medically acceptable body composition ratios are related to:

1. Lower risk for respiratory infections.
2. Lower blood pressure.
3. Less risk for atherosclerosis.
4. Lower risk of some forms of cancer.
5. Less risk for developing adult-onset diabetes.

Medically acceptable body composition ratios lengthen the lifespan and improve the quality of life. Good body composition has psychological and social benefits. Finally a good body composition ratio enhances physical movement and achievement in athletic activities. People with poor body composition are likely to develop various health problems.

Glandular disorders are the cause of 5% or less of all obesity. Medical treatment is necessary for glandular disorders. Children can develop extra fat cells, termed *hyperplasia*. These children seem to have a greater propensity to become obese as adults. When the *size* of fat cells increases, in obese adults, it is termed hypertrophy. Teens (13–18) who are too fat are at greater risk for heart problems and cancer than their lean peers.

One's basal metabolic rate (BMR) can change. When the BMR decreases, calorie intake must decrease also or the activity level has to increase to prevent a gain in fat weight. In short, when caloric intake exceeds caloric expenditure over time, obesity is the result. Exercise uses calories, which makes it valuable in losing weight.

---

[13] *Badminton Today,* p. 104.

Medically related obesity must be addressed by a physician. Medical check-ups should also be a first step for anyone over age 40 who is considered a high risk for some conditions. Otherwise, the solution to reducing fat from one's body is simple in principle. Some people, however, have difficulty carrying out the necessary steps. The following suggestions will help in reducing body fat and achieving a better body composition ratio.

1. Exercise! No single factor is more responsible for obesity than the lack of physical exercise.
2. Decrease your intake of total calories and calories from dietary fat.
3. Utilize (burn) more calories than you eat. Exercise combined with dietary restriction is the most effective method of reducing fat. *Just* dieting or *just* exercising is not as effective as both.
4. Do exercises that can be sustained for relatively long periods.
5. Exercise at moderate intensity, which suppresses the appetite.

Measuring Body Composition

Various methods are used to measure body composition.

1. *Skinfold measurements* are taken using skinfold calipers. Various sites on the body are used, depending on the particular protocol. A formula is used to determine or calculate the percent fat for an individual. The measurement produces an estimate.
2. *Hydrostatic weighing* involves the subject being immersed in a tank of water. This requires special equipment and someone trained to figure the fat percentage. This is the most reliable method.
3. Other measurements related to obesity are:
   a. Waist-to-hip circumference ratio: an index for determining risk and disease associated with fat and weight distribution, calculated by dividing the waist measurement by the hip measurement. A chart provides a classification of risk.
   b. Height-weight measurements: Charts are consulted to determine the recommended weight, by gender for various heights and body frame size.

   c. The Body Mass Index (BMI): The index formula is:

$$\frac{\text{body weight in kilograms}}{(\text{height in meters})^2}$$

Divide the subject's weight in pounds by 2.2 to determine weight in kilograms. Multiply the height in inches by .0254 to determine height in meters. The final calculated result is compared to a chart for classification of risk.

Value of Body Composition for Pickle-Ball

The value of having a good body composition ratio of lean-to-fat tissue can be summed up in the following.

1. Low body fat enables better flexibility and better performance.
2. Low body weight reduces the stress and strain on muscle groups, particularly the lower body and back.
3. Low body weight allows the player to be quicker on the court because he or she is carrying less fat around the court.
4. Excessive body weight leads to quicker fatigue and loss of effectiveness.

Specific Body Composition Needs for Pickle-Ball

1. The average or tall player can use the longer levers of the arm to produce the needed force to produce strokes with proper speed.
2. Less body fat to allow quicker movement on the court.

Review Questions

1. Each component of fitness is _____ of the other and requires specific measurements and procedures to develop and maintain.

2. Fitness is _____-specific.

3. Flexibility is critical to the overall prevention of _____.

4. _____ activities help condition the heart and lungs for the quick bursts of energy needed for long rallies.

5. _____ activities increase the endurance necessary for long matches.

6. Long rallies in Pickle-Ball demand both _____ and

   _____ endurance.

7. The component of _____ allows you to hit the ball harder.

8. Strong _____ and _____ muscles are necessary to move quickly to every shot.

9. Excessive body weight, or _____, will cause undue fatigue and players will lose effectiveness quickly.

10. Low body weight will reduce the stress and strain on _____ groups.

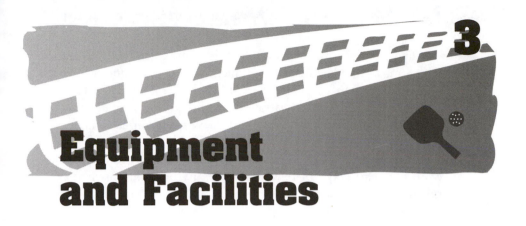

Equipment
and Facilities

The game of Pickle-Ball is played with a paddle and a plastic perforated ball on a small court divided by a low net. Pickle-Ball is a relatively inexpensive sport, and equipment is not prohibitive to purchase by anyone. Figure 3.1 illustrates Pickle-Ball equipment.

PADDLES

The paddle is made of durable 7-ply hardwoods. Hardwood paddles are ideal for teaching paddle control and directing the plastic ball to the opponent's court. Wood paddles provide the best paddle control for hitting the plastic ball to a specific location on the opponent's court. The United States of America Pickleball Association, Inc. indicates that the paddle may be constructed of any suitable material.

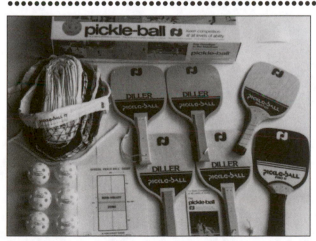

Diller, Master, and Pro II Pickle-Ball paddles. Complete set includes four Diller/Master paddles, six Pickle-Balls, heavy-duty net, and official Pickle-Ball rules.

PHOTO COURTESY OF PICKLE-BALL, INC.

FIGURE 3.1

The paddle's overall length should not exceed 15½ inches, with a maximum head width of 8 inches and a maximum weight of 13 ounces. Most Pickle-Ballers think the ideal weight is 10 to 12 ounces. A short cord is attached to the butt of the handle for safety and should always be around the wrist during play. Figure 3.2 shows the parts of the paddle.

The head of the paddle is distinctly squared-off rather than oval. the head may not be strung, nor any perforations or texturing materials allowed on the surface. Thus, surfaces with sandpaper, holes, or glued granules are prohibited.[1]

BALLS

This sport's projectile is a plastic sphere with small holes (Figure 3.3). The maximum diameter of the ball is 3 inches.[2] The Dura 56 ball is a seamless plastic polyball that has been specially designed and manufactured for Pickle-Ball use. This rotationally molded ball can be used indoors or outdoors on any hard surface. This unique ball will provide truer flight and extend the durability of the ball over other plastic balls.

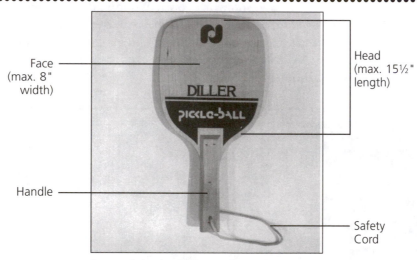

Face
(max. 8"
width)

Head
(max. 15½"
length)

DILLER

ᑭꞮᴄᴋᴌᴇ-ᴅᴀᴌᴌ

Handle

Safety
Cord

Parts of the paddle.

FIGURE 3.2

---

[1] Dick Squires, *The Other Racquet Sports* (New York: McGraw-Hill, 1978), p. 235.
[2] Squires, p. 235.

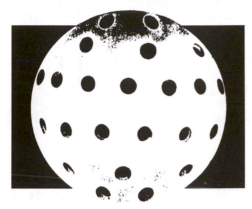

Pickle-Ball.

FIGURE 3.3

NETS

The official heavy duty Pickle-Ball net may be used for play. Many physical educators lower their badminton nets to a height of 3 feet as a means of converting their badminton courts to Pickle-Ball courts.

COURTS

The official rules of Pickle-Ball set the dimensions of the court to be 20 feet by 44 feet, which also happen to be the dimensions of the badminton doubles court. The same size court is used for both singles and doubles. The court is divided by a net 36 inches high on the sides of the court and sloping to 34 inches in the middle.

The non-volley zone is the area 7 feet on each side of the net. The center line divides the area behind the non-volley zone into two equal service courts. The short service line on the official badminton court is 6 feet 6 inches from the net. This line may be used for the non-volley zone when Pickle-Ball is played on the badminton court in the gymnasium. Figure 3.4 depicts the court. There should be space of at least 3 to 5 feet beyond the ends and 1 to 2 feet beyond the sides to provide for adequate player movement.

A portable tournament set is ideal for elementary programs or school physical education programs that do not have heavy-duty volleyball or badminton standards (Figure 3.5). This set

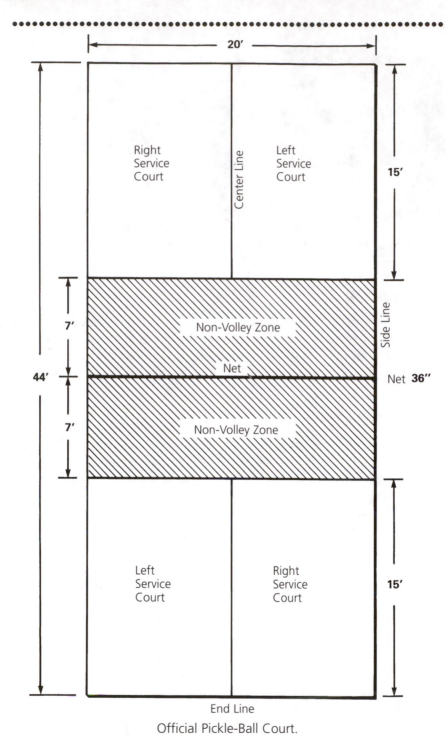

Official Pickle-Ball Court.

FIGURE 3.4

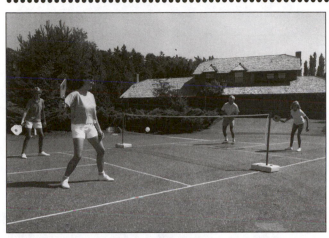

Portable
Pickle-Ball Sets.

*PHOTO COURTESY
PICKLE-BALL, INC.*

FIGURE 3.5 ●●

can be set up in 10 minutes on any hard surface, indoors or outdoors on a playground. This set contains two water-fillable base
standards, two net posts, four wooden paddles, three balls, one
lightweight net, and chalk for lines.

All Pickle-Ball equipment and publications may be obtained
from: Pickle-Ball, Inc. 801 N.W. 47th St., Seattle, WA 98107;
phone: 206-784-4723 or FAX: 206-781-0782.

·············Review Questions

Completion

1. The Pickle-Ball paddle has a maximum head width of _____

   and should not exceed _____ in length.

2. _____; _____ or _____
   are prohibited on the head of the paddle.

3. The maximum diameter of the official Pickle-Ball is _____.

4. The outer dimensions of the court for Pickle-Ball doubles and singles

   are _____ (the same).

5. The Pickle-Ball net should be _____ high at

   the sides and slope to _____ in the middle.

6. The non-volley zone is the area _____ feet on each
   side of the net.

7. There should be a space of at least _____
   beyond the ends of the court to provide for adequate player
   movement.

•••

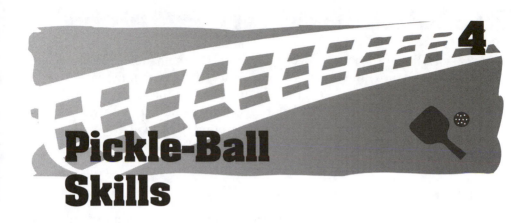

Pickle-Ball Skills

The beginner's goal in Pickle-Ball is to develop consistent control of the paddle on the ball. This requires the ability to regulate the speed and direction of the ball.

The basic strokes needed to play Pickle-Ball are the forehand and backhand drives, the serve, and the forehand and backhand volleys. The paddle must be firmly held throughout the stroke, especially upon contact with the ball. Between strokes, however, the hand must be relaxed.

GRIPS

Eastern Grip

The Eastern grip is used when stroking the ball on the dominant or paddle side of the body. This hand position is sometimes called the "handshake grip" (see Figure 4.1).

To position your hand for this grip, hold the paddle in the non-dominant hand with the hitting surface perpendicular to the floor. Slide the hand onto the paddle as you would to shake hands with someone. The right forefinger is spread slightly away from the other fingers to help hold the paddle more efficiently. The thumb should be wrapped around the handle to make contact with or lie close to the inside of your middle finger. The paddle should be lying across the palm and fingers with the thumb and index finger forming a V on the top of the paddle handle.

When the ball comes to the nondominant side of the body, the hand shifts position on the handle. With the hitting surface perpendicular to the floor, place the palm on top of the handle with the wrist slightly to the left. Spread your fingers comfortably around the handle, again extending the index finger. The knuckle of the index finger rests on top of the handle. This is a quarter turn counterclockwise to your left. The thumb may be placed at a 45° diagonal across the back of the handle. Some think the thumb should be straight up the handle toward the head of the paddle to gain better leverage. This will give additional support and act as a brace against the impact of the ball in the backhand drive (see Figure 4.2).

Western Grip

The Western grip is used primarily to impart topspin on the ball during the forehand drive. To obtain the Western forehand grip, simply lay the paddle on the floor, then pick it up by the handle. The hand will be approximately an eighth turn to the right of the Eastern forehand. The Western backhand grip is basically the same as the Eastern but involves a considerable shift of the hand.

Continental Grip

The Continental grip is midway between the Eastern forehand and backhand. No change is made from the forehand to the backhand, thus offering a distinct advantage in an exchange of rapid strokes at the net when volleying (see Figure 4.3).

Table 4.1 shows some common grip errors and how to correct them.

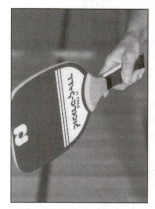

FIGURE 4.1
Eastern Forehand.

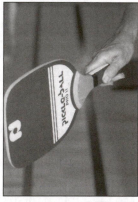

FIGURE 4.2
Eastern Backhand.

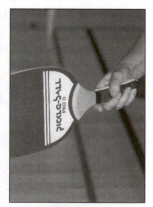

FIGURE 4.3
Continental.

TABLE 4.1••
Common Grip Errors and How to Correct Them.

GRIP ERROR	CORRECTION
1. Choking the paddle	1. Move hand down and explain value of using total length of paddle.
2. Holding the paddle too tightly	2. Spread fingers around the handle; stress relaxing between strokes.
3. Extending first finger behind the paddle head, resulting in limited wrist action	3. Review correct hand position; extend fingers around the handle.

••

⊕ READY POSITION

The efficiency with which you return the ball is dependent on how you prepare to stroke the ball. The ready position allows you to move in any direction to return the opponent's shots. The feet should be spread shoulder-width and the knees slightly flexed with the weight on the balls of the feet. The back should be fairly straight and inclined slightly forward, head up, and eyes on the opponent. The paddle should be held in front of the body about waist level and pointed at the opponent. Hold the paddle with a relaxed forehand grip (see Figure 4.4).

••

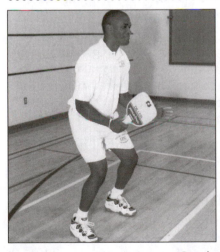 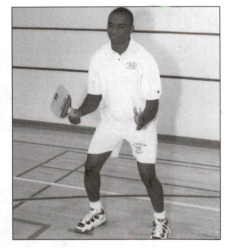

Ready Position.

FIGURE 4.4 ••

Table 4.2 shows some typical errors in the ready position and how to correct them.

TABLE 4.2••
Common Errors in Ready Position and How to Correct Them.

ERROR IN READY POSITION	CORRECTION
1. Locking the knees	1. Flex the knees slightly.
2. Not squaring the body with the net	2. Square the body to the net.
3. Holding down the paddle by the legs	3. Hold the paddle in front of the body, at least waist high, ready to play the ball.
4. Placing the weight back on the heels	4. Place the weight on the balls of the feet.
5. Standing with the feet an improper distance apart	5. Place the feet about shoulder-width apart.

••

⊜ COURT COVERAGE

Good footwork means moving into position in a way that enables you to take an efficient hitting stance, even under difficult conditions. An efficient stance is sometimes "open," sometimes "closed." In an open stance, the outside foot is closer to the net than the inside foot and the body is facing the net. In a closed stance, the forward foot is several inches nearer the sideline than the back foot.

Good movers make adjustments in their steps. They adjust the size, the speed, and the timing so they can take the stance that is best or possible on each hit. This requires speed of foot, agility, mobility, body control, and balance.

Two concepts underlie good footwork.

1. The player moves to a spot to await the ball in flight only after an opponent has executed a return shot. The player avoids shifting weight forward in anticipation of a short return until the opponent has hit the ball.

2. The player takes the last step before contacting the ball with the paddle foot, if possible. This step is important for maintaining balance and proper shift of weight on the stroke and for the return to ready position.

For baseline play, try to be in a ready position just in front of the middle of the baseline as your opponent meets the ball. This puts you in the best position to move in the various directions required to return the ball. To reach balls 8 to 10 feet to the side, cross over quickly with the left foot for a ball going to your right (forehand) or with your right foot for a ball going to your left (backhand). Try to get set to hit with your body weight on the back foot. This lets you step in with the forward foot as you swing. Move with little steps so you will be better able to adjust them and because they give more starting speed than big steps. Start your backswing as soon as you begin to move, and adjust the amount of time you have to make it.

The player may shuffle to reach a ball 4 or 5 feet away. To shuffle to the right, push off with the left foot while raising the other and moving it several inches to the right. Place your weight on the right foot, and bring the left foot up alongside it. A quick shift of weight to your left foot will permit another push-off and shuffle to the right. After your second shuffle, pivot on your right foot and swing your left foot across to place your body in a hitting position.

Shuffle when only two shuffles will let you reach the ball. Three or more are awkward and slow. Return to center position by a shuffle in the opposite direction.

You can move back from the net in much the same way. If two shuffles will get you into position, you can move that way. Start by pivoting on your left foot, and at the same time swinging your right foot backward. Then shuffle to the backcourt. In moving back to play a short lob, go back far enough to let the ball come down into your hitting area so you can play the ball conveniently.

On deep lobs you will probably have to turn and run to get into position, draw your right foot back and cross the left one over the right, and start running toward the baseline. While running back, look toward the net at the ball.

To get away from a ball hit close to your right side, move your right foot back and to your left while making your backswing. Then step toward the left net post with your left foot as you make the forward swing.

Short balls in both the forehand and backhand corners should be retrieved by running toward the corner and ending with the dominant leg forward, directly under the paddle. This position allows you to stretch and reach the balls more efficiently.

DRIVES

Forehand Drive

The forehand drive is a natural hitting movement, similar to batting a baseball (see Figure 4.5). The ball is played after it has bounced once from the paddle side of the body. If the ball is allowed to bounce twice before it is returned, a fault is called, using the term "not up." From the ready position, pivot toward the sideline and simultaneously draw the paddle back at waist

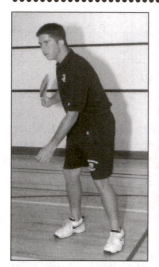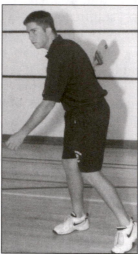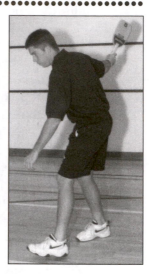

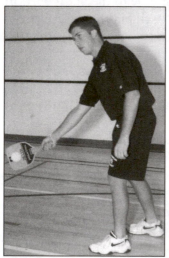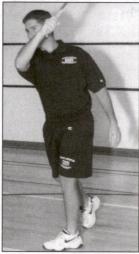

Forehand Drive.

FIGURE 4.5

level. This must be a complete pivot with the feet, hips, and shoulders all facing the sideline. Beginners often fail to do this movement fully. The body weight shifts to the rear foot.

TABLE 4.3••
Common Forehand Errors and How to Correct Them.

FOREHAND ERROR	CORRECTION
1. Hitting the ball too long	1. The face of the paddle may be open or tilted too far up. Tilt it downward. You may be letting the ball drop back down to the floor before you play it. Adjust your timing.
2. Hitting the ball too short	2. Step into the ball and shift your weight with each shot. Be sure to have a good follow-through, with the paddle finishing well in front of the body.
3. Consistently hitting ball to the right (right-handers) or to the left (left-handers)	3. Position the body facing the sideline, and contact the ball even with the front foot. The paddle should be parallel to the net on contact. Do not let the wrist "give" on impact with the ball.
4. Consistently hitting the ball to the left (right-handers) or to the right (left-handers)	4. Position the body facing the sideline, and contact the ball even with the front foot. The paddle should be parallel to the net on contact. Do not let the wrist "give" on impact with the ball.
5. Loss of power as ball is contacted late behind the body	5. Contact the ball off the forward foot; rotate the left side of the body to the net.
6. Not maintaining eye contact with the ball throughout the complete stroke	6. Maintain eye contact with the ball as it leaves the opponent's paddle until the ball has left your paddle on the return stroke.
7. Dropping the head of the paddle rather than bending the knees	7. Keep the paddle head even with the wrist, and bend the knees to play low balls.

••

You are now ready to begin the forward swing of the paddle to contact the ball. Step toward the net with a shift of weight from the rear foot to the front foot as the paddle moves forward and upward. The paddle face should be flat at the instant of contact. This upward movement of the paddle will impart slight topspin, which will help keep the ball in the court. The forward knee, as you step, must bend slightly to absorb the shifting weight from the rear to the front foot. The grip should tighten on the paddle just before contact with the ball. The paddle should meet the ball at a point directly in front of the forward foot.

After contact, the paddle should continue in the intended direction of the ball for as long as possible. The arm should swing across the body toward the target, reaching as far as possible. The forward foot now has most of the body weight, and the forward knee is bent to retain balance and to help in a fast return to the ready position.

Backhand Drive

Basically the backhand drive involves the same mechanics as the forehand, but it is executed on the opposite side of the body — the non-paddle side (see Figure 4.6). From the ready position, pivot toward the sideline and simultaneously draw the paddle back at waist level. The main difference between the backhand and forehand positions is the shoulder pivot. For the backhand, the shoulders are turned more than they are for the forehand. At the completion of the backswing, you should be looking over your shoulder to see the approaching ball. The paddle is swung completely around the body to the opposite hip level, and the grip is changed on the handle. The arm and paddle are closer to the body than in the forehand drive. On the pivot, the hips turn toward the sideline and the weight shifts to the rear foot. The forward foot steps across so the back is half-turned toward the net.

As the forward swing begins, the weight is shifted forward by pushing from the rear foot and bending the forward knee. The uncoiling of the hips and shoulders starts the forward swing of the paddle. The paddle moves forward and upward with the face flat at the instant of contact. The hand and paddle move away from the hip in the direction of the oncoming ball. The grip should tighten on the paddle just before contact with the ball. The ball is contacted directly in front of the forward foot.

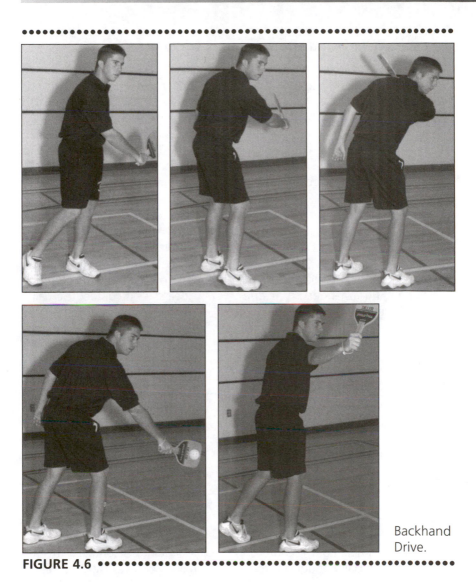

Backhand Drive.

FIGURE 4.6 •••

A complete follow-through and finish are necessary to give power and direction to the ball. After contact, the paddle should continue in the intended direction of the ball as long as possible. At the finish, the paddle is at shoulder level or higher. The opposite arm is extended away from the body for balance. The weight is transferred to the front foot, and the forward knee is slightly bent. You are ready to return to the ready position. Some typical backhand errors appear in Table 4.4, along with some ways to correct them.

TABLE 4.4••
Common Backhand Errors and How to Correct Them.

BACKHAND ERROR	CORRECTION
1. Hitting the ball too long	1. The face of the paddle may be open or tilted too far up. Tilt the paddle downward. You may be letting the ball drop back down to the floor before you play it. Adjust your timing.
2. Hitting the ball too short	2. Step into the shot and shift your weight with each shot. Be sure to have a good follow-through with the paddle finishing well in front of the body.
3. Consistently hitting the ball to right (right-handers) or to the left (left-handers)	3. Position the body facing the sideline, and contact the ball even with the front foot. The paddle should be parallel to the net on contact. Do not let the wrist "give" on impact with the ball.
4. Consistently hitting the ball to the left (right-handers) or to the right (left-handers)	4. Position the body facing the sideline, and contact the ball even with the front foot. The paddle should be parallel to the net on contact. Do not let the wrist "give" on impact with the ball.
5. Loss of power as the ball is contacted late behind the body	5. Contact the ball off the forward foot; rotate the right side of the body to the net.
6. Not maintaining eye contact with the ball throughout the complete stroke	6. Maintain eye contact with the ball as it leaves the opponent's paddle until it has left your paddle on the return stroke.
7. Dropping the head of the paddle rather than bending the knees	7. Keep the paddle head even with the wrist, and bend the knees to play low balls.
8. Not changing the grip	8. Rotate the hand on the handle to the backhand grip.

••

An important factor in directing your shots is to control the angle of the paddle face at impact with the ball. The desired return angle of the ball will be determined by the height of the ball at the moment of impact.

1. If the ball is below the level of the net, the paddle face must be opened to allow the ball to rise up over the net on the return flight (see Figure 4.7).

2. When the ball has bounced higher than the top of the net, the paddle face should be closed to help keep the ball down on the return flight over the net (see Figure 4.8).

3. A flat face should be used to return a ball parallel to the floor and just over the top of the net (see Figure 4.9).

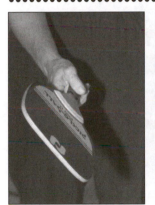 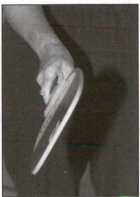 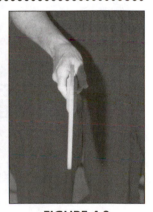

FIGURE 4.7
Open Face.

FIGURE 4.8
Closed Face.

FIGURE 4.9
Flat Face.

BALL SPIN

The kind and amount of spin on the ball are determined by the position of the paddle and the direction in which the paddle is traveling upon contact with the ball. Understanding spin and the effect it has on the flight and bounce of the ball will assist you in varying your stroke production and in preparing for groundstroke and service returns. When you are able to control ball spin and can also play the spinning ball after it bounces, you will be well on your way to achieving a well-rounded game.

A spinning ball moves in the direction of its rotation. A ball that is spinning forward tends to drop; a ball spinning backward tends to rise; and a ball spinning sideways tends to curve left or right.

To produce topspin, start the paddle from a position behind and below the ball with either a slightly closed or flat face. Move the paddle forward and upward through the ball, keeping the face perpendicular to the intended line of flight. Continue upward after contact, finishing high and in front of your body.

Topspin provides a greater margin of error because the shot crosses the net higher than the typical flat shot and drops sharply within the baseline. This permits the player to hit harder while still retaining control.

The backspinning ball, after being hit, turns away from the direction in which it is moving. To impart backspin, the paddle

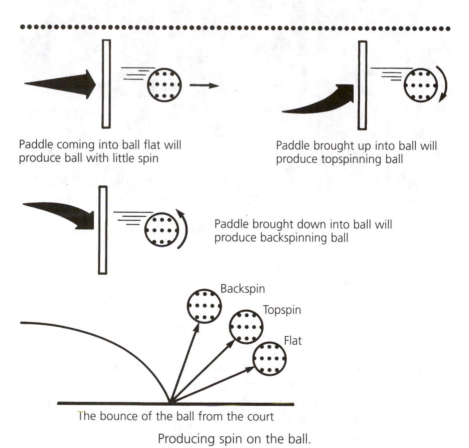

Paddle coming into ball flat will produce ball with little spin

Paddle brought up into ball will produce topspinning ball

Paddle brought down into ball will produce backspinning ball

Backspin

Topspin

Flat

The bounce of the ball from the court

Producing spin on the ball.

FIGURE 4.10

starts from a position behind and above the ball, strikes the back side, and continues down and through the ball (high to low).

To control the amount of spin, open the face of the paddle. The greater the high-to-low angle and the slant of the face, the greater is the backspin.

Backspin causes the ball to rise slightly after contact, producing a floating type of flight. When the ball hits the floor, it loses much of its forward momentum. It may either die or bounce sharply upward, depending on the amount of spin and the angle at which the ball approached the floor. Backspin is especially good for low volleys and drop volleys.

SERVES

To put the ball in play, you must use an underhand motion, and the paddle must pass below the waist. You must hit the ball in the air and keep one foot behind the backline when serving (see Figure 4.11).

You are not allowed to bounce the ball, then hit it. Use a forehand grip for the service. The receiver must allow the serve to bounce before returning it.

The purpose of the serve is to put the ball in play. We emphasize that the serve be an underhand motion with the paddle face contacting the ball below the hip. We do not promote

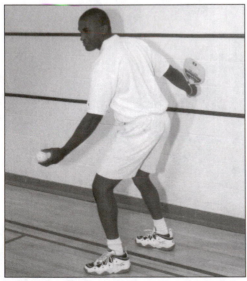

Feet position on serve.

FIGURE 4.11

"hard winning serves" as in tennis. The goal of the serve is to promote rallies between opponents.

Drive Serve

A hard, deep drive serve will keep the opponent at the baseline and on the defense (see Figure 4.12). A poor return of service will allow the server to take the attacking position. To execute this serve, take a forward stride position with the nondominant foot forward and at least one foot behind the end line. The feet should be comfortably apart with the weight on the back foot. The paddle arm is extended away from the body, and the paddle is held behind you about waist height with the wrist in a

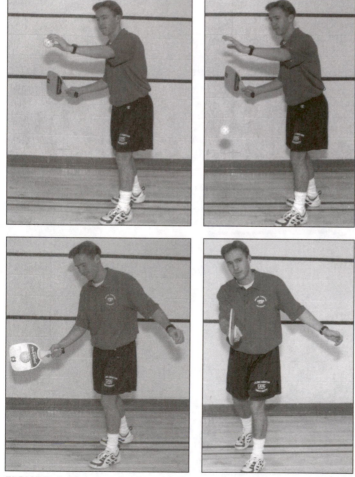

Drive Serve.

FIGURE 4.12

cocked position. The ball is held out in front of the body about waist height.

As you drop the ball well out in front of your body, the paddle swings down and forward. The weight is shifted from the back to the front foot as the body is rotated to the left so it faces the direction of the ball's flight. The paddle arm is straightened at point of contact with the ball. Quickly after contact, the wrist and forearm are pronated as the paddle is swung upward. Follow-through of the paddle is about shoulder height as the pronation takes place.

Lob Serve

The lob serve can be used for a change of pace and will also keep the receiver at the baseline on the defense (see Figure 4.13). The ball will also have a high bounce and be difficult to return effectively. The preparation for this serve is exactly the same as for the drive serve. The point of contact of the paddle with the ball is higher, and the paddle is made to lift the ball high and deep to about one foot inside the end line. The forearm and wrist do not pronate, but follow through straight forward to about head height. Table 4.5 lists some common errors in the lob and drive serves and how to correct them.

TABLE 4.5••
Common Serve Errors and How to Correct Them.

DRIVE SERVE ERRORS	CORRECTIONS
1. Hitting the ball in a low trajectory into the net	1. Contact the ball sooner, and lift the ball over the net.
2. No control over ball direction	2. Follow through in the direction of the desired flight.
3. Poor ball release, resulting in poor serve	3. Concentrate on dropping the ball, then swinging the paddle.

LOB SERVE ERRORS	CORRECTIONS
1. Serving too high and shallow	1. Stress wrist and forearm flexibility. Bring paddle high on follow-through.
2. No control over ball direction	2. Follow through in the direction of the desired flight.
3. Poor ball release, resulting in poor serve	3. Concentrate on dropping the ball, then swinging the paddle.

••

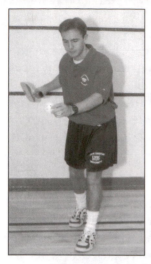
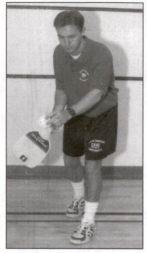
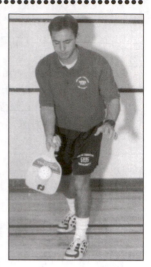
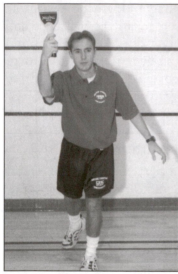

Lob Serve.

FIGURE 4.13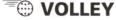

VOLLEY

To have an aggressive offense, you must have a net game that develops around the volley. The volley is used to play the ball before the bounce and from a position just behind the non-volley zone of the court. Singles offense calls for a strong volley, as it is the finishing stroke for many points. In doubles the volley is even more important, because the strategy of the game is to play from the net. To be effective, the volley must be made from above the net, where it can be hit downward for a winner. If the ball is contacted below net level, it becomes a defensive shot and must be hit upward to clear the net. This may become a put-away for your opponent.

The grips used for the volley are the same as for the drives — the Eastern forehand and the Eastern backhand. The Continental grip may be used for quick rallies at the net when there is not time to change grip between forehand and backhand exchanges.

The basic volleying position is about 1 foot behind the non-volley zone. The ready position is the same as for the ground-strokes, except the paddle is held about eye level.

On the volley you are trying to stop the progress of the ball rather than slam the ball back over the net. The volley has little or no backswing. For a rapidly approaching ball, you may have time for only a slight turn of the shoulders (see Figure 4.14).

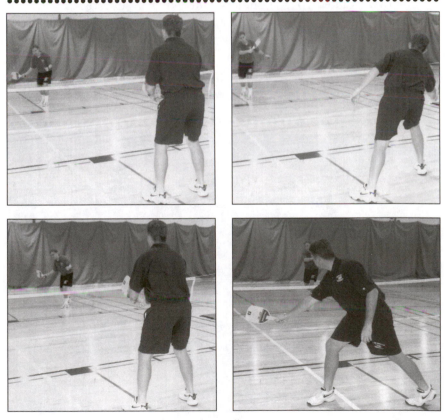

The Volley.

FIGURE 4.14

Usually, the shoulder turn is combined with a step toward the ball with the lead foot (see Figure 4.15). Meet the ball in front and to the side of your body; do not let it come to you. Weight should be transferred to the forward foot with a slight bend in the knee to absorb the weight. You should squeeze the grip just before impact with the ball to help keep the wrist firm at contact. Keep your eyes on the ball, and meet it in the center of the paddle so its impetus will not turn the paddle in your hand.

In the volley there is little follow-through in the direction of the ball. Also, the rules state that the player cannot follow through with a step into the non-volley zone after volleying the ball. If this happens, it is a fault.

If the ball is several feet to one side, meet it by taking a cross-over step; step across your body with the left foot to hit a ball on the right side, and vice versa for the left side. This cross-over rotates your shoulders and extends your reach with the paddle.

When you are forced to volley the ball from below the level of the net, the stroke will be primarily defensive. Tilt the paddle

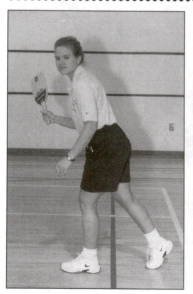
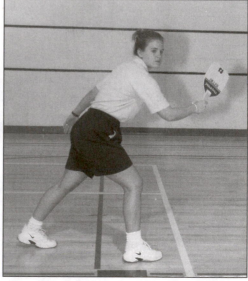

Volley Step Across.

FIGURE 4.15

face back to hit this volley, and lift the ball over the net. Bend the knees and get down to the ball, and keep the paddle higher than the handle (see Figure 4.16).

When the ball is hit directly at you, take it with a backhand stroke (see Figure 4.17). Push your elbow out to the side, lower the paddle, and pull it across horizontally in front of you to block the ball and send it back over the net. Table 4.6 lists some common errors in volleying and ways to correct them.

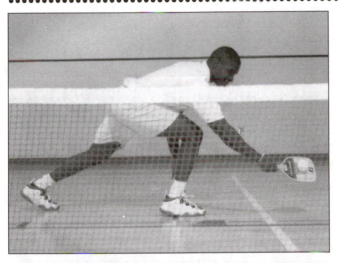

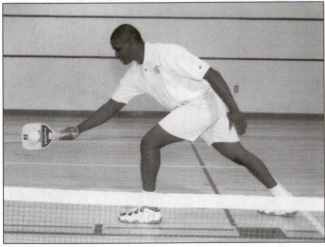

Defensive Volley.

FIGURE 4.16 ●●●

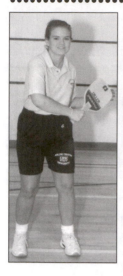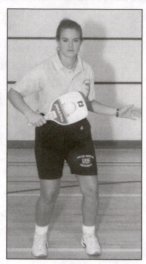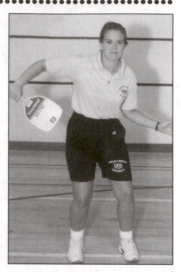

Volley ball hit directly at you.

FIGURE 4.17 ••

TABLE 4.6••
Common Volley Errors and How to Correct Them.

VOLLEY ERROR	CORRECTION
1. Ball going too long	1. Shorten the amount of backswing, and punch the ball. Also, limit the amount of follow-through
2. Hitting ball too easily	2. Meet the ball in front of your body. Step to the ball; do not let it come to you. Contact the ball in the center of the paddle.
3. Ball going too high	3. Bend the knees and get down to the ball. Keep the paddle head above or even with the handle.

 LOB

When your opponent rushes the net you can use the drive down the line, a short crosscourt, or a lob. Lobs are of two types: offensive and defensive. The offensive lob is used to force the net player back to the baseline into a less advantageous position. The defensive lob usually provides time for the player drawn out of position by an opponent's placement to recover and get back into position on the court.

The lob begins the same way as the drive, whether on the forehand or the backhand side. Grip, stance, and backswing are identical; this can be good deception for the aggressive player.

The difference between executing the drive and the lob lies in the angle of the paddle face when contact is made with the ball as the paddle moves in a low to high path through the forward swing and the high follow-through. Let the paddle do the work for you in the lob, lifting the ball high and forward to the opposite baseline (see Figure 4.18 and 4.19).

The offensive lob should be over your opponent's head, just out of reach of his paddle. The best lob will require your opponent to return with a backhand, usually the player's weakest stroke.

Just as the offensive lob is kept fairly low, the defensive lob must be hit fairly high. A good defensive lob will go about 25 feet in the air and land about 1 to 2 feet inside the baseline, giving you time to recover your position on the court. Table 4.7 delineates some common lob errors and how to correct them.

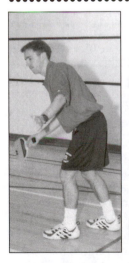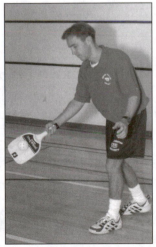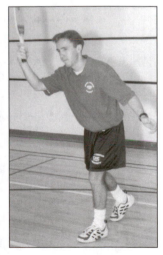

Forehand Lob.

FIGURE 4.18 •

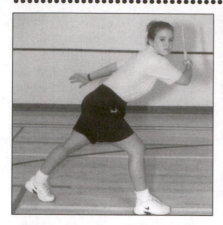
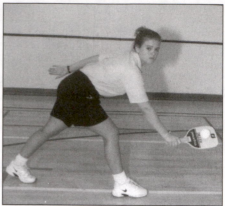
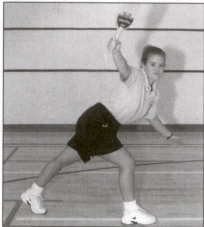

Backhand Lob.

FIGURE 4.19 ●●

TABLE 4.7●●
Common Lob Errors and How to Correct Them.

LOB ERROR	CORRECTION
1. Hitting balls too short	1. Get set sooner. Use the arm more, and drive up and through the ball. Follow through fully. Carry the ball up with the paddle.
2. Mis-hitting ball often	2. Get into position as soon as possible. Watch the ball carefully as it hits the paddle.
3. Improper angle of paddle face	3. Open up the paddle face to get height and distance.

●●

SMASH

The smash is used to hit the ball downward with authority and placement from midcourt prior to the bounce. The forehand grip is used, and timing of the contact is important to play the ball correctly. You must get into position under and in back of the ball with your body under control. As you move into position to play the ball, move the paddle into position behind your head, with your elbow pointing slightly upward, causing the paddle to drop down to the floor. The non-paddle hand is pointed up to the ball to help you keep your eyes focused on it. Your back should be bent slightly backward, your body should be angled slightly sideways to the net, and the weight should be on your rear foot.

The paddle changes direction at the beginning of the forward swing and is thrown up and forward to meet the ball as the elbow leads the action. The wrist follows the elbow upward, and the arm extends toward the ball.

The ball is contacted about 1 foot in front of the dominant shoulder and as high as possible with a flat paddle. A wrist snap sends the paddle ahead of the wrist at contact and helps keep the ball down in the court. Continue the follow-through down and to the side of the body. Finish with the dominant side foot stepping forward to maintain your balance; recover quickly to the ready position for the next shot (see Figure 4.20). Table 4.8 lists some common smash errors and how to correct them.

DROP SHOT AND DROP VOLLEY

Drop shots and drop volleys add excitement and flavor to the game and are necessary for you to be a complete player. To be successful, they require a soft touch and knowledge of when and when not to use them.

A baseline player may be drawn to the net, a slow player may be caught deep in the court, and an opponent may be tired out by tactical use of the drop shot. This shot is usually attempted when the player is in a good position on the court — about mid-court.

The drop shot is executed after the ball has bounced. It is gently hit with underspin so it will just barely clear the net and land in the non-volley zone close to the net. Deception is important to success of this shot, so the preparation and stroke must look like any groundstroke until the moment of contact. The

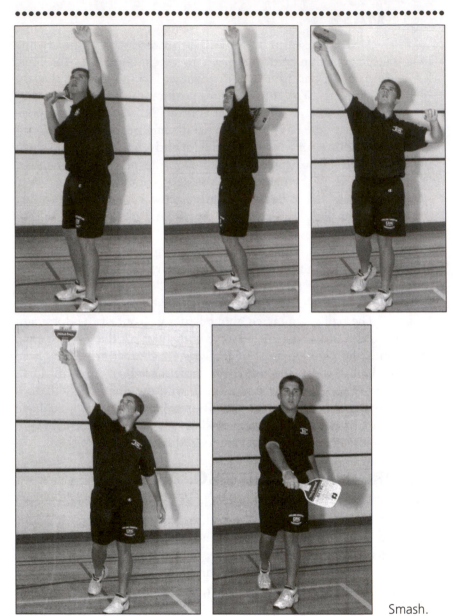

Smash.

FIGURE 4.20

ball is hit to the side and in front of your body. Just before contact, open the face of the paddle to brush the back and underside of the ball, giving it underspin to slow down its motion. The follow-through continues downward and forward.

TABLE 4.8••
Common Smash Errors and How to Correct Them.

SMASH ERROR	CORRECTION
1. Ball going too long	1. The ball is hit too early or above the head. Contact the ball out in front of the body. Tilt the paddle face more toward the floor.
2. Driving ball into net	2. Contact the ball high and drive it forward and downward with powerful wrist and forearm rotation. Follow through to the spot of intended flight.
3. Little power with smash	3. Arch your back and throw the paddle upward into the ball. Rotate your upper body, shift your weight, and contact the ball with powerful wrist and forearm rotation.

•••

The drop volley is used when the player is at the net. This is also a surprise shot and should be used carefully. It is hit with underspin so it barely clears the net and lands short in the opponent's non-volley zone. Deception is again important, and preparation and backswing should be similar to your normal volley. Move the paddle head downward and forward, opening the paddle face to brush the underside of the ball. Upon contact with the ball, relax the wrist slightly and let the paddle head give a little to deaden the impact of the ball, causing it to lose some of its speed. This action will result in a short volley. Angle the ball away from your opponent if possible. A good rule to follow is not to use the drop volley if the ball can be put away with a deeper volley.

HALF-VOLLEY

The half-volley is a defensive shot when the ball is hit immediately after the bounce. The ball has usually been hit directly at your feet in the backcourt, and you do not have time to get into position to drive the ball. Also, you may be caught when approaching the net and do not have time to volley the return.

You bend your knees and place the paddle so the ball provides the power for the return as it rebounds from the floor.

The height of this shot is controlled by the angle of the paddle face. From the backcourt, the face is more closed to prevent the ball from going too high over the net on the return. As you approach the net, the face is opened to raise the ball over the net.

Review Questions

True or False

T   F   1. When using the forehand grip, the thumb extends up the top plate of the handle of the paddle.

T   F   2. In the forehand grip, the forefinger is extended directly up the handle of the paddle.

T   F   3. In executing a forehand or a backhand drive, the follow-through should be in the direction of the intended flight of the ball.

T   F   4. In hitting a forehand drive, the ball should be contacted when it is opposite the right foot, if right-handed.

T   F   5. As part of the preparation for a forehand drive, the left-handed player should turn toward the right-hand sideline.

T   F   6. In the backhand grip, the palm of the paddle hand should be facing the ground.

T   F   7. In hitting a backhand drive, the player should look over the right shoulder at the oncoming ball.

T   F   8. In hitting a drive, the beginner should look at the desired target on the other side of the net.

T   F   9. When serving, the ball should be hit with the paddle arm fully extended.

T   F   10. In returning a lob with an overhead smash, proper body position is directly behind the intended point of contact.

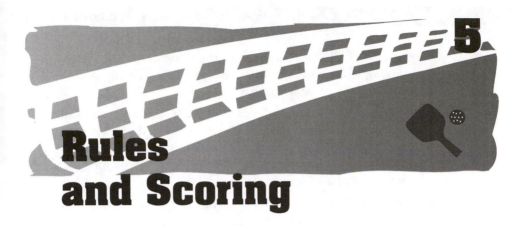

Rules and Scoring

The originators of the game developed the rules of Pickle-Ball during the first months and year of play. The beginning rules depended heavily on badminton. Various changes occurred throughout the game's evolution. The following rules for Pickle-Ball are presented as they appear in the Official Pickle-Ball Rules (reprinted by permission of Pickle-Ball, Inc.).

OFFICIAL PICKLE-BALL RULES

1. Court — The size of the court is 20' x 44' for both doubles and singles. The net is hung at 36" on ends, and hangs 34" in the middle. When laying out a court, allow adequate space at each end and sides of the court boundary lines for player movement (3 to 5 feet on ends and 1 to 2 feet on sides). However, it should be noted that many families play Pickle-Ball with little or no back and side court and enjoy the game (see Figure [3.4], Official Pickle-Ball Court).

2. Serve — Player must keep one foot behind the back line when serving. The serve is made underhand. The paddle must pass below the waist. The server must hit the ball in the air on the serve. He is not allowed to bounce it, then hit it. The service is made diagonally cross court and must clear the non-volley zone. Only one serve attempt is allowed, except if the ball touches the net on the serve and lands in the proper service court. Then the serve may be taken over. If the server attempts to serve the ball, and misses the ball with the paddle, it shall count as an attempted serve. At the start of each new game, the first serving team is allowed only one fault before giving up the ball to the opponents. Thereafter, both members of each team will serve and fault

before the ball is turned over to the opposing team. When receiving team wins the serve, the player in the right-hand court will always start play.

3. Volley — To volley a ball means to hit it in the air without first letting it bounce. All volleying must be done with the player's feet *behind* the non-volley zone line. NOTE: It is a fault if the player steps on or over the line on the volley follow through (see Figure 5.1).

4. Double Bounce Rule — Each team must play its first shot off the bounce. That is, the receiving team must let the serve bounce, and the serving team must let the return of the serve bounce before playing it. After the two bounces have occurred, the ball can be either volleyed or played off the bounce (see Figure 5.2).

5. Fault —

   a. Hitting the ball out of bounds;

   b. Not clearing net;

   c. Stepping into the non-volley zone and volleying the ball;

   d. Volleying the ball before it has bounced once on each side of the net as outlined in rule 4.

6. Scoring — A team shall score a point only when serving. A player who is serving shall continue to do so until a fault is made by that team. The game is played to 11 points;

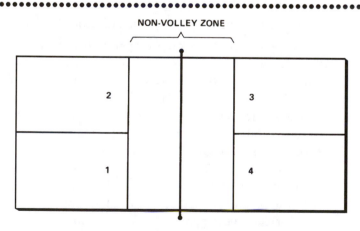

Court showing non-volley zone.

FIGURE 5.1

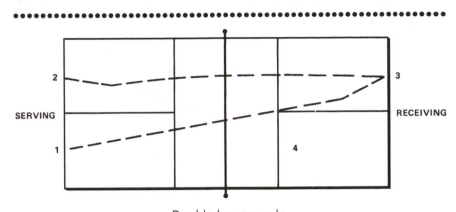

Double-bounce rule.

FIGURE 5.2

however, a team must win by 2 points. A match will be the best of three games unless otherwise agreed-upon.

7. Position of players for doubles at start of game (see Figure 5.3).

8. Determining serving team — Players may toss a coin or rally the ball until a fault is made. Winner of the toss or rally has the option of serving first or not serving first.

9. Doubles play —

    a. Player in **right-hand** court (1) serves diagonally across court to receiver (3) in opposite **right-hand** court (see Figure 5.4). The ball must clear the non-volley zone and

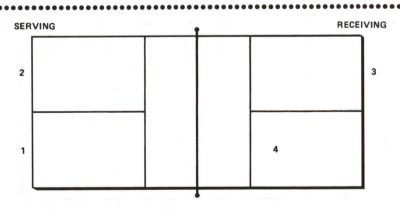

Position of doubles players at start of game.

FIGURE 5.3

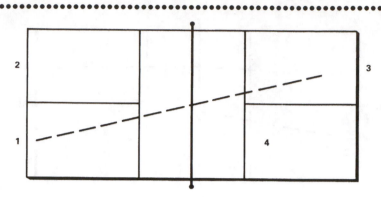

Serving to receiver in doubles play.

FIGURE 5.4

land in the **right-hand** serving court. The receiver (3) must let the ball bounce before returning the serve. Serving team must also let the return bounce before playing it. (RULE #4 — Double Bounce Rule). After the two bounces have occurred, the ball may then be either volleyed or played off the bounce until a fault is made.

b. If the fault is made by the receiving team, a point is scored by the serving team. When the serving team wins a point, its players will switch courts and the same player will continue to serve (see Figure 5.5).

c. The player not returning the serve, who is in the up position at the net, may not inhibit or intimidate the server by

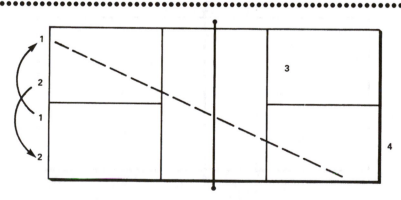

Switching courts after serving team wins point.

FIGURE 5.5

waving his paddle or leaning over into the receiving court. The server may ask the net player to refrain from these actions. These actions are considered unsportsman-like conduct.

When the serving team makes its first fault, players will stay in the same court and the second partner will then serve. When they make their second fault, they will stay in the same courts and turn the ball over to the other team. Players switch courts only after scoring.

10. Singles Play — All rules apply with the following exception: When serving in singles, each player serves from the **right-hand** court when his score is 0 or an even number, and from the **left-hand** court when the score is odd-numbered.

11. General Tips —

    a. Both members of the serving team should be back near the baseline at the time of the serve so that neither will forget to let the first returned ball bounce before returning it (see Double Bounce Rule).

    b. After the ball is in play, lobbying it over the opponent's head can be effective strategy.

    c. A ball landing on any line is considered good.

    d. If a player sees that the ball is going to land in the non-volley zone, and he or she is going to let it bounce, the player may move into the zone before it bounces but must let it bounce before returning it (see Figure 5.6).

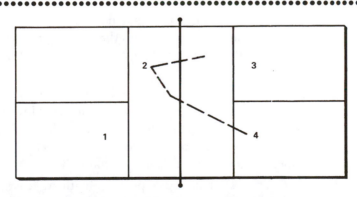

Receiver position in non-volley zone.

FIGURE 5.6

e. The player who starts the game in the right-hand court score 0) will always be in the right-hand court when this team's score is 2, 4, 6, 8 and 10.

f. The hand below the wrist is considered part of the paddle, and shots off any part of it are good.

ADDITIONAL RULES FOR THE SERIOUS PLAYER

1. If a player serves out of turn, or from the wrong service court, or receives in the wrong court, and *his or her side wins the rally,* it shall be a "let," providing that such "let" be claimed before the next succeeding service is delivered. If a player standing in the wrong service court takes the service, and *his or her side wins the rally,* it shall be a "let," provided that such "let" be claimed before the next succeeding service is delivered.

   If in any of the above cases the side at fault loses the rally, the mistake shall stand and the players' position shall not be corrected during the remainder of the game.

   Should a player inadvertently change sides when he or she should not do so and the mistake not be discovered until *after the next* succeeding service has been delivered, the mistake shall stand, a "let" *cannot be claimed,* and the players' position shall not be corrected during the remainder of that game.

2. The server may not serve until his or her opponent is ready, but the opponent shall be deemed to be ready if a return of service is attempted.

3. If a player is playing a ball that has bounced in the non-volley zone and he or she touches the net with the paddle or any part of the body, it shall constitute a fault for that player.

4. A service fault occurs when the server swings the paddle with the intent of striking the ball but misses. However, the server may toss the ball into the air and then catch it or allow it to fall to the court without penalty, so long as he or she does not attempt a delivery of that ball.

5. The server must take up a position with at least 1 foot behind the baseline without touching that line, and between an imaginary extension of the center line and the sideline.

Both feet must be inside the imaginary line extensions or a fault shall be called on the server.

6. Only the player served to may receive the service, but should the ball touch, or be struck by, his or her partner, the serving side scores a point.

7. A fault is called when a player is hit by the ball whether he is standing inside or outside the court boundaries.

8. A ball seemingly going out of bounds must be allowed to hit the floor out of bounds. It is a fault to catch the ball and claim that it was going out.

9. Before beginning the game, the players must decide who will serve first from which end of the court. A coin may be tossed to allow the winner to make the first choice, and the other player the remaining choice. If there are identifying marks on each side of the paddle, it may be spun by placing the head on the ground and spinning it like a top. Before the spinning paddle falls to the ground, the other player will call out one of the identifying marks on the paddle, hoping it will fall with that side up.

   The player winning the toss may choose or require the opponent to choose from among the following: (1) to serve or to receive, or (2) to begin play on a specific end of the court. The player not making the original choice has the choice of the remaining options. It must be noted that if one player chooses end of the court, the opponent is *not* automatically required to serve. Instead, the opponent has the remaining choice — to serve or receive.

   Usually, the player who wins the toss elects to serve first. This is because many players consider serving first to be a psychological as well as a physical advantage. However, if one side of the court is considered to be the best because of background or some other factor, the winner of the toss may find it more advantageous to select side rather than serve.

   Any player wanting an interpretation of the rules as established by the United States of America Pickle-Ball Association, Inc. may write to: Sid Williams, 3015 No. Pearl St. Apt. #H122, Tacoma, WA 98407.

·······················Review Questions

True or False

T   F   1. The official Pickle-Ball court has the same dimensions as a badminton singles court.

T   F   2. Pickle-Ball singles and doubles are played on the same size court.

T   F   3. The Pickle-Ball net is the same height in the middle of the court as on the sides.

T   F   4. Both feet must be kept behind the back line when serving in Pickle-Ball.

T   F   5. The serve is made with an underhand motion, with the paddle below the waist.

T   F   6. The server is not allowed to bounce the ball, then hit it on the rebound.

T   F   7. The serve is taken over any time the ball touches the net while passing over it.

T   F   8. At the beginning of a doubles game, both players on a team will serve before the opponents are allowed to serve.

T   F   9. The doubles player in the right-hand court will always serve first for his or her team.

T   F   10. Hitting the ball before it bounces is a volley.

T   F   11. A player may not volley the ball while standing in the non-volley zone.

T   F   12. It is legal for a player to step into the non-volley zone immediately after volleying the ball.

T   F   13. Each team must play its first hit off the bounce.

T   F   14. The Double Bounce Rule means that the ball may be allowed to bounce twice before a player returns it.

T   F   15. The person serving will serve until the receiving team makes a fault, and then the partner will serve, except on the first service for the team.

T   F   16. When the score is odd, the doubles partners will be in the court in which the team did not begin.

T   F   17. In singles, when the server's score is even, he or she will be serving from the right-hand court.

T   F   18. A player may move into the non-volley zone and play a ball if he or she lets it bounce before returning it.

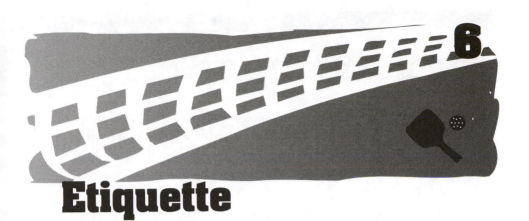

Etiquette

As in any sport, the official rules of Pickle-Ball govern only the technicalities of the game. Many years of playing racket or paddle games have established unwritten customs and traditions now in use. The following are guidelines for proper Pickle-Ball conduct:

1. Dress according to the rules established by the center or school where you play.

2. Be on time for your game. The only thing more rude than being late is not showing up at all.

3. Do not distract other players by walking behind their court during play. Wait until the point is finished and then hurry to your court.

4. Always know your opponent. If you have never met, introduce yourself in a friendly manner.

5. Take a brief warm-up period (approximately 5 minutes) before each game. Both players should take all practice serves before playing any points.

6. Before serving, make sure your opponent is ready.

7. The server is responsible for keeping score and announcing the score clearly to the opponent before serving each point. The server's score should be given first.

8. Do not return a serve that is obviously out. Let is go past you or block it into the net so it will not be in the way. Returning serves that are out is a discourteous action in Pickle-Ball.

9. Make calls on your side of the net fairly, giving your opponent the benefit of the doubt on close calls. A ball should be considered good unless it is clearly seen to be out.

10. Retrieve balls from adjacent courts by waiting until the point is over and then politely saying "thank you" or "ball, please."

11. Return balls from adjacent courts by waiting until play has stopped and then tossing them softly and accurately to the nearest player.

12. If a ball enters your playing area, stop play immediately and play a "let."

13. Recognize good play by your partner or opponent. Keep in mind, however, that Pickle-Ball is a game of concentration. Talk only when it pertains to the game or changing sides.

14. After each point, quickly collect all balls on your side of the court. Hustling after stray balls makes the game go much faster.

15. Control your feelings on the court. Abide by the rules, and always display sportsmanlike conduct.

16. Replace cracked balls quickly as possible.

Review Questions

Completion

1. The only thing more rude than being late for a Pickle-Ball match is

   _____.

2. You have been given court two for your game. There is a game in progress on court one of the gymnasium. When should you move to your court to begin play?

3. When should practice serves be taken?

4. What two things should the server do before serving?

   a.

   b.

5. Whose score should be given first when calling out the score?

6. What two actions can be taken with a serve that is out?

   a.

   b.

7. What should you *never* do with a serve that is not good?

8. A ball should be considered good unless _____.

9. How should you go about retrieving a ball from an adjacent court?

    a.

    b.

10. How should you return a ball from an adjacent court?

    a.

    b.

11. What should you do if a ball enters your court during the point?

●●●

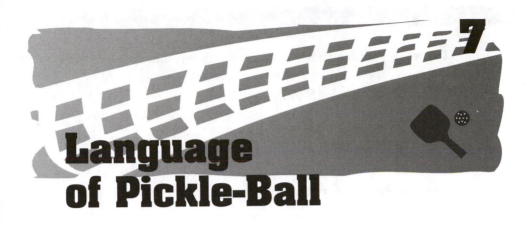

Language
of Pickle-Ball

The language of Pickle-Ball has evolved from the games of badminton and tennis. The player should be able to converse about the game with knowledge and command of the terminology.

Ace. A serve that the receiver cannot get to and that scores a point for the server; a winner.

All. A tied score, as in 6-all.

Approach Shot. Usually a groundstroke hit deep into opponent's court, allowing hitter to go to the net.

Backcourt. The area around the baseline.

Backhand. A stroke used to play the ball on the non-paddle side of the body.

Backspin. Spin applied to the ball by hitting down behind it, causing it to spin the opposite direction of its flight.

Change of Pace. The strategy of changing the speed of the ball from stroke to stroke.

Chop. A movement in which the paddle is drawn down and under the ball, imparting backspin to the ball.

Crosscourt Shot. Placing the ball from one side of the court across the net to the side diagonally opposite.

Deep. A shot that lands within the court near the baseline.

Doubles. A game played between two teams of two players — two men, two women, or a man and a woman in mixed doubles.

Down-the-Line Shot. A ball that travels low over the net and parallel to the sideline.

Drive. A ball hit after the bounce with medium speed so that it will travel to the end of the opposite court.

Drop Shot. A ball hit softly with backspin so that it just clears the net and lands very close to it in the non-volley zone.

Drop Volley. A ball volleyed with underspin so it barely clears the net and lands short in opponent's non-volley zone.

Earned Point. A point won by the player's skill rather than opponent's error.

Error. A point lost because of poor play, not caused by opponent. Many more points are lost on errors than are won on placements or on earned points.

Even Court. The right-hand court, because when serving from this court, an even number of points have been played in the game. Partners will be on the side of the court on which they started the game.

Face. The hitting surface of the paddle. In a *closed face,* the hitting surface is turned down toward the floor. In an *open face,* the hitting surface is turned up toward the ceiling. In a *flat face,* the hitting surface is perpendicular to the floor.

Fault. A served ball that does not land within the proper service court; sometimes refers to an illegal serve or return.

Foot Fault. An illegal service; usually the server fails to keep one foot behind the end line.

Forcing Shot. Usually a fast, deep, and well-placed attacking shot designed to force a weak return or an error by your opponent.

Forehand. A stroke used to play the ball on the paddle side of the body.

Game. Completed when one side has won 11 points, with a 2-point lead.

Game Point. The point that wins the game for the player or team scoring it.

Gherkin. A rally which, if won by the server, ends the game. Also called **game point.**

Groundstroke. Hitting the ball after it has bounced.

Half-volley. Usually a defensive stroke in which the ball is contacted immediately after it begins to rise from a bounce.

Head. The part of the paddle used to hit the ball.

Let. A point that must be replayed.

Let Serve. A ball that hits the top of the net on the serve and lands in the correct service court; must be replayed.

Lob. A high, arching shot over the reach of the net player that lands near the opponent's baseline.

Match. Best of three games unless otherwise agreed upon.

Match Point. The point that wins the match for the player or team scoring it.

Mixed Doubles. Team composed of male and female partners.

Net Game. Strategy in which the player advances to the net to use the volley and smash to end the point.

Non-volley Zone. The area 7 feet on either side of the net; the player may not step into this area or onto the non-volley zone line to *volley* a ball. It is also a fault if the player steps into this area or on the non-volley zone line on the follow-through of a *volley*.

Not Up. Allowing the ball to bounce twice before returning it; a fault.

Odd Court. The left court, because when serving from this court, an odd number of points has been played. Partners will be on the side of the court on which they did not start the game.

Smash. An overhead stroke used to put the ball away.

Passing Shot. Sending the ball quickly over the net past an opponent's reach.

Pickle. A rally that, if won by server, ends the match; also called "match point."

Poach. Usually in doubles, the net player moving across the court to cut off a ball that normally would be played by the partner.

Put Away. A ball hit so well that the opponent cannot return it; a winner.

Rally. Continuation of play after the serve in which the players keep the ball in play for several strokes.

Rush the Net. A style of play in which the player hits an approach shot and takes the net to be in a better position to win the point.

Serve. Underhand stroke used to put the ball in play at the beginning of each point.

Singles. A game played between two players.

Spin the Paddle. At the beginning of a game, spinning a paddle so it will land flat on the floor. The non-spinner calls which side the paddle will fall on. The winner of the spin may choose to serve or receive first, or which court he or she wants. The loser makes the remaining choice.

Topspin. Spin applied to the ball by bringing the paddle up behind it, causing the ball to spin in the direction of its flight.

Volley. Hitting a ball before it bounces.

Review Questions

True or False

T   F   1. When a player returns a drive so well that the opponent cannot get to it, it is called an ace.

T   F   2. When both players have 10 points, it is called 10-all.

T   F   3. An approach shot is when the net player hits a volley deep to the backcourt.

T   F   4. Change of pace is not good strategy to use, as it will be confusing to the doubles partners.

T   F   5. A down-the-line shot travels diagonally from one side of the court across the net to the opposite side of the court.

T   F   6. A ball hit before the bounce with medium speed so it will travel to the end of the opposite court is a drive.

T   F   7. A drop shot just clears the net and lands in the non-volley zone.

T   F   8. A point won by the player's skill rather than an opponent's poor play is called an error.

T   F   9. Many more points are lost on errors than are won on placement or on earned points.

T   F   10. The even court is the right-hand court, because an even number of points has been played when serving from this side.

T   F   11. In doubles, the partners will be in the court in which they started the game when their score is odd.

T   F   12. A foot fault occurs when the server fails to keep both feet behind the baseline when serving the ball.

T　　　F　　　13. A game is completed when one side has won 15 points, with a 2-point lead.

T　　　F　　　14. A half-volley occurs when the ball is stroked with the paddle immediately after the ball has bounced.

T　　　F　　　15. A ball low over the net just out of reach of the net player is called a lob.

T　　　F　　　16. A high, arching shot over the reach of the net player that lands near the opponent's baseline is called a half-volley.

T　　　F　　　17. A passing shot is a ball hit quickly over the net just out of reach of the opponent.

T　　　F　　　18. When the net player moves back from the net position to allow the partner to play the ball, it is called poaching.

T　　　F　　　19. Rushing the net is a style of play in which the player returns every ball as quickly as possible.

T　　　F　　　20. Spin applied by bringing the paddle up under the ball, causing it to spin in the direction of its flight, is called topspin.

PICKLE-BALL TERMS

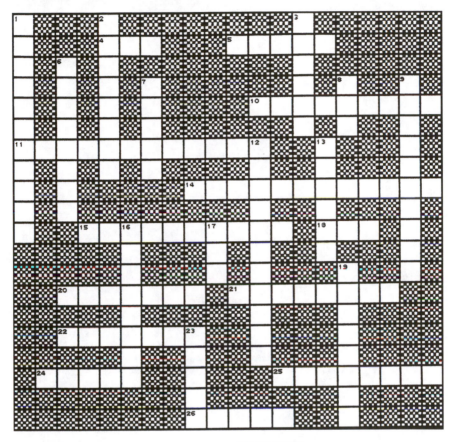

ACROSS CLUES

4. When the score is tied
5. Point lost because of poor play
10. Right court in singles
11. Hitting ball after bounce
14. Deep groundstroke allowing hitter to go to the net
15. Ball contacted immediately after it begins to rise from bounce
18. Point that must be replayed
20. Paddle goes up behind ball and ball spins in direction of flight
21. Stroke on paddle side of the body
22. Point that wins the game
24. Ball hit after the bounce that goes to end of the court
25. Ball hit after bounce with backspin that barely clears net and lands in non-volley zone
26. Net player cuts off ball at the net that would be played by partner

DOWN CLUES

1. Send ball over the net out of opponent's reach
2. Stroke used to play ball on non-paddle side of body
3. Hit the ball before it bounces
6. Left court in singles
7. Overhead stroke used to put the ball away
8. Serve that cannot be played by receiver; a winner
9. Ball volleyed with backspin so it drops just over the net
12. Point won by player's skill
13. Point that wins the match
16. Serve hits top of net and lands in correct service court
17. High shot that lands near opposite baseline
19. Hitting down on ball so it spins in opposite direction of flight
23. Ball bounces twice before it is returned; a fault

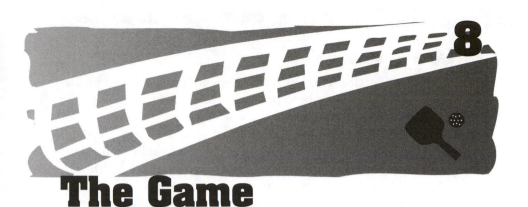

The Game

When you first start to play the game, you are concerned primarily with keeping the ball in the court and getting the feel of the short paddle and the low bounce of the ball — especially if you are an experienced tennis player. During these games, try to (1) hit most balls deep into the opponent's court, (2) hit most balls to the opponent's weakest side (usually the backhand), and (3) move the opponent around the court by hitting the ball from side to side.

As you gain experience in Pickle-Ball, you should begin to adopt a strategy that fits your own personal skills. You must build your strategy around four aspects of the game: service, return of service, net play, and baseline play. A discussion of these aspects of the singles and doubles game follow, given for the right-handed player.

THE SINGLES GAME

The Service

The most advantageous positions from which to serve are near the center line when serving into the even court, and a couple of feet from the center line for the odd court. Before you serve, decide how and where you are going to serve the ball. Three general placements for the serve are: (1) deep to the far corner in both courts, (2) down the middle, close to the center line, and (3) directly at the receiver.

Vary the pace and the placements of your service so your opponent is not able to guess how and where you are going to serve the ball. Do not try to serve the ball too close to the lines; give yourself some room — about 1 foot inside the lines of the service court.

Return of Service

Return of service is an important element in the game of Pickle-Ball that all players should practice. The receiver must allow the ball to bounce before returning it.

The receiver should assume a position of readiness: head up, hips and knees flexed slightly, weight on the balls of the feet. The feet should be spread a little more than shoulder-width with the paddle held in front of the body at about shoulder height.

Your position on the court must allow freedom to move wide for serves hit in the far corners or toward the center line for serves hit up the middle.

The distance you stand from the net is determined by the speed of your opponent's serve. For a fast, hard serve, you must take a deep position behind the baseline so you can prepare for the return. Also for the fast serve, you must stroke the ball with a firm wrist and utilize the power the server has already applied to the ball.

Most serve returns should be hit deep to the server's forehand or backhand corners. Hard serves that come wide to the forehand in the even court and wide to the backhand in the odd court are easily returned with a deep down-the-line shot. Slow and short serves can be returned easily with crosscourt shots, as they allow time to play the ball and give a better angle for shot placement. Any service return deep to the opponent's backhand will often force the server to return with a weak short shot, which you can put away for a winner, or a placement that will allow you to take the net.

Net Play

Because of the small size of the Pickle-Ball court, net play becomes important in the singles game. A player can control the pace of the game from the net and gain a distinct advantage. A player, however, cannot step into the non-volley zone, on the follow-through of a volley. A player can move into the area if the ball has already bounced but should retreat back to a legal position to play the next ball.

A player has to advance to the net carefully, and the advance must be well planned. It should always follow a forcing shot that has put your opponent on the defensive. Most opportunities to rush the net follow short returns by your opponent. After forcefully returning the short ball, continue to a position about 2 feet behind the non-volley zone.

A deep placement to one of the corners, usually the backhand, will prepare you for your advance to the net. As you move to the net, drift toward the side of your placement to bisect the angle of the return. The wider your shot, the more you must crowd the sideline.

Following an approach shot, you must move to the net quickly, keeping your paddle in readiness on the way. As you move to the net, watch your opponent and as he or she is about to make the return, pause and be ready to move in any direction for the ball. If you are caught in a poor net position, you may be forced to hit a defensive volley or a half-volley. If this happens, put the volley deep down the middle to cut down the angle of return.

When at the net, be aggressive. Put the ball away. Put the ball out of your opponent's reach, or when you have him or her on the run, put the ball in the area of the court that the opponent just left. A good return of a short lob is directly at the feet of your opponent, which is difficult to play.

Your presence at the net gives you a psychological advantage, too. It may force your opponent into self-forced errors on routine balls.

Baseline Play

Baseline play is basic to Pickle-Ball. Without it, the net rusher will have difficulty going to the net. Strategy from the baseline begins with simply keeping the ball in play. Let your opponent make the error.

When playing from the baseline, you must learn to keep the ball deep. Any ball you return short will allow your opponent to be aggressive and take the net. This does not mean you have to hit the ball as hard as possible — just keep it as close to the baseline as possible.

When returning balls from the baseline, you must expect a large portion of them to be returned, and you will have to move about the court fairly well. To allow yourself maximum court coverage capability, you must return to a position on the court near the center of the baseline after each shot.

Baseline strategy involves, first of all, running your opponent from side to side. This will cause him or her to anticipate moving from side to side, and you can then surprise your opponent and hit to the same side twice in a row. You may also hit balls to one side of the court and then send a ball deep to the opposite corner.

If your opponent has a definite weak side, play balls to that side. He or she will become frustrated upon missing several shots in a row. The aggressive player takes advantage of this frustration.

When your opponent seems to play both sides of the court equally well, you will want to play the ball keep down the middle of the court. This will lessen the opponent's crosscourt possibilities from both sides of the court.

When players stay on the baseline and do not come to the net, they usually are weak net players or just do not like the fast exchange that happens there. The smart player will try to bring this opponent up to the net with a drop shot inside the non-volley zone and make him or her do what that player does not want to do. After bringing the opponent to the net, send him or her deep again with a lob to the baseline. This alternating strategy will tire your opponent more quickly than running him or her from side to side.

THE DOUBLES GAME

Many doubles games seem to be mass confusion on the court, with no planning. Most games will be with different partners and do not afford you much time to plan strategy. Some basic doubles tactics, however, will lead to exciting, well-played games.

The team that has control of the net will, in most instances, win the game. The offense in doubles is built around the serve, volley, and smash. The lob is the major defensive stroke.

The receiving team begins with one player at the net, and the receiver will want to follow the return to the net even with the partner. Because of the Double-Bounce Rule, both members of the serving team must remain in the backcourt until the ball has bounced twice; they must let the ball bounce in their court once before going to the net to volley the ball. The serving team must be prepared to lob its first return if the opponents are aggressive at gaining the net. The serving team must play the ball down the middle to confuse the opponents.

The Service

The game of doubles is based on positioning. The receiving team has an advantage over the serving team because the receiver's partner is already at the net at the beginning of each point. The net player has the responsibility of guarding the sideline, but he or she should move to the center to cut off any weak return.

The appropriate position at the net is about 2 feet behind the non-volley zone and about 3 feet inside the sideline. The net player must not slowly drift toward the center of the court during a rally, giving the opponents an opening down the line for a winner.

The server should take a position halfway between the center line and the sideline, or slightly more to the sideline. The server's partner should be halfway between the center line and the sideline on his or her side of the court, and on or slightly behind the baseline. The serving team must remain in the back-court until it has played the ball after it has bounced once (Double Bounce Rule).

Generally, serves should be deep to the receiver's backhand corner, possibly causing a weak return of service. An occasional serve should go to the forehand to keep the receiver guessing.

Because only one service is allowed to put the ball in play, the server should be more concerned for accuracy than power. Drive and lob serves should be mixed, but not in a noticeable pattern.

Return of Service

The return of service in doubles is important. It may help the receiving team gain control of the net, as the return must be allowed to bounce on the serving side of the court.

The depth and strength of the service determines how deep the receiver will stand. The receiver should be ready to play either a forehand or a backhand serve.

The receiver's partner should take a position about 2 feet behind the non-volley zone and 3 feet inside the sideline. The receiver should come to the net, even with his or her partner, on return of service, to put the team on the offense.

Return of service has several possibilities.

1. Directly to the partner of the server, if he or she is too close to the net to not let the ball bounce before playing it.

2. Directly at the server's feet, forcing a weak return.

3. A hard drive down the middle, creating confusion as to who will play the ball, especially if the serve was close to the center line. For a deep serve in the outside corner of the even court, a down-the-line return is good because it will be to the opponent's backhand.

Be sure to notice if your opponents are right- or left-handed, as this will greatly affect the placement of returns.

Net Play

The total strategy for doubles is for both partners to gain possession of the net. The receiving team has the advantage to begin each point and must protect it with good return-of-service shots.

The serving team's best opportunity to gain the net is to force the receiving team members away from the net with a well-placed, over-the-head lob on the first return of the ball after it has bounced. The lob should be hit either to the backhand corner or up the middle to create confusion between the two partners as to who will return the shot. A team that has been pushed away from the net will many times lob the ball back, hoping to regain the net position.

On its first hit after the serve the serving team may also try to gain the net with a well-placed drop shot just over the net into the non-volley zone. The opponents must let the ball bounce in the non-volley zone before hitting it and will probably have to hit the ball up on the return. This will allow a possible put away by the opposing team, which has come to the net following the drop shot. This well-placed drop shot may also cause the opponents to foot fault by trying to play the ball before it bounces and stepping into the non-volley zone on the volley or the follow-through.

The basic net position for both partners is about 2 feet behind the non-volley zone and midway between the sideline and the center line. They should always be even with each other (see Figure 8.1).

The smash should be hit at the feet of one of the opponents, or crosscourt when the sharply angled shot is available. A simple strategy is to *hit the ball where the opponents are not.*

If one of the net players is drawn off or to the side of the court to play a ball, the partner should drift slightly in that direction to maintain maximum court coverage. When a lob is made over the head of one player, *both* should retreat from the net to a defensive position. They should maintain a side-by-side position throughout the rally.

The player who can play the ball with a forehand should play balls hit between the two partners. When a lob is hit up the middle over the head of the net players, the partner who can get to it with a forehand return should take the ball. When the ball is lobbed over the head of one player, the other player usually has the best chance of retrieving the shot. The players will

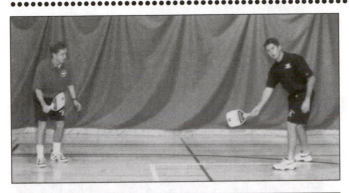

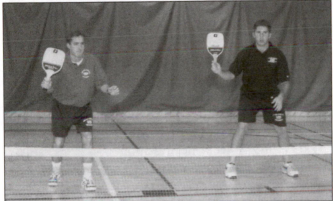

Taking control of the net.

FIGURE 8.1 •••

switch sides, with the net player dropping back to the other side, and continue play. If only one player moves back to return a deep lob and decides to let it bounce, the net player must also retreat to a defensive position in the backcourt.

Poaching is the action of one player moving over to cut off a ball that would normally be played by the partner. An experienced player may anticipate where the opponent's shot will come and drift in that direction before the ball is on its way. This movement leaves the sideline open for a passing shot by the opponent, so it must not become habitual for the net player.

Baseline Play

All play from the baseline should be in preparation for an advance to the net. This is usually accomplished by a lob or by a low crosscourt return. When both opponents are at the net, a hard-hit drive between the partners will often result in a winner because it creates confusion as to who will play the ball. Many times a drive directly at a net player will result in a point because that player does not react quickly.

PICKLE-BALL DOUBLES STRATEGY

Pickle-Ball involves strategies that include lobbing, overhead slamming, passing drive shots from the baseline, and fast volley exchanges at the net. The key strategy to remember is that the team that reaches the front court in a net volley position first will be in the best position to win the point. Again, the most effective position of play is when both players on the same team are side-by-side in the attack position 2 feet behind the non-volley zone line.

Player Position on the Court

The serving team will be side-by-side on the baseline in a defensive position ready to return passing drive shots, drop shots, and overhead smashes. The serving team must stay back until the ball has bounced once on its side prior to moving forward to the net volley position. The receiving team will have the player not receiving the serve in the net volley position.

The player receiving the serve should play 1–2 feet behind the baseline to anticipate the deep serve of the opposing team. The receiving team player should hit a deep return of service shot and move forward to the net volley position side-by-side with the partner. This is the ideal attack position for the receiving team as both players are in the *best* position to win the point (receiving team in net volley position hitting overhead slams and drop shots, and serving team in defensive position back on the baseline attempting passing, drive shots, offensive lobs deep to the baseline, and drop shots that fall into the non-volley zone).

Shot Selection — Receiving Team on Offense

The receiving team in the net volley position may utilize the following shots to win back the serve:

1. Overhead smashes down the middle of the court or angled toward the sidelines.

2. Drop shots clearing the net and landing in the non-volley zone (a player may move into non-volley zone before ball bounces, but the player must let it bounce before returning it). Drop shots can be effective as the serving team players are back in a side-by-side baseline position prepared for

overhead smashes. They must rush forward and hit an "off-balance" shot, which is usually a "put-away" overhead slam or volley by the receiving team.

It is to the receiving team's advantage while at the net volley position to return all possible shots on the fly, not on first bounce. If the receiving team lets an offensive lob bounce, it may relinquish the net volley position, as the serving team will seize this opportunity to move forward and gain the net volley position while the receiving team retreats to the defensive position on the baseline.

Shot Selection — Serving Team on Offense

Both serving-team players will be side-by-side, one foot behind the baseline. The ideal serve is hit hard and deep diagonally to the receiving team player. The advantage of a hard-hit deep serve is that the receiving player who returns service will have greater difficulty moving forward and "getting set" in the net volley position.

The serving team can take advantage of this deep serve by hitting a short drop shot that will land in the non-volley zone just in front of the on-rushing receiving player, who is moving forward to join the partner at the net volley position.

Remember — the serving team must let the return of service shot bounce once on its side prior to moving forward to the attack position. If the receiving team is set at the net volley position, the serving team can utilize the following shot selection:

1. Passing, drive shots toward the receiving team player who is moving forward after hitting the return-of-service shot to establish the net volley position.

2. Lobbing shots deep to the receiving team's baseline. High, deep lobs drive the receiving players back to the baseline, and many times the receiving team will let the ball bounce, thinking the ball will fall out of bounds, beyond the baseline. At this point, the serving team seizes the opportunity to move forward to take the net volley position away from the receiving team.

3. "Dink" or Drop-Shot. An effective "dink" or drop shot is when the ball lands in the non-volley zone and the receiving team is unable to hit the ball on the fly without faulting (hitting ball on fly in non-volley zone). Once the receiving team lets the ball bounce in the non-volley zone, the serving team

rushes to the attack position. Now the serving team has created a situation in which it is on equal terms at the net volley position with the receiving team, therefore, creating fast volley exchanges at the net. This short drop-shot strategy creates fast and furious volley exchanges between all four players stationed at the net volley position.

Again, Pickle-Ball is a sport where shot placement, steadiness, patience, and tactics have far greater importance than brute power and strength.

Mixed Doubles

Although the game usually becomes more relaxed and friendly with mixed doubles, this is not always true. Fierce competition may still be present.

There are no rules as to how mixed doubles partners should serve or receive. This is a matter for the partners to decide before the game. The stronger player might want to begin the game in the odd court to have the forehand covering the middle of the court.

All suggestions for regular doubles play apply to mixed doubles. The fact that men and women can compete against and with each other makes Pickle-Ball an appealing game for all concerned.

.....................Review Questions

Completion: The Singles Game

1. The singles serve into the even court should be made standing

   _____.

2. When serving to the odd court in singles, the server should stand

   _____.

3. Three general placements for the serve are:

   a. _____

   b. _____

   c. _____

4. How can you keep your opponent from being able to anticipate where you are going to serve?

   a. _____

   b. _____

5. In the ready position, where should the paddle be?

   _____

6. The distance you stand from the net to receive service is determined

   by _____.

7. Most serve returns should be hit _____.

8. What will a player often expect when returning a serve deep to the

   opponent's backhand court? _____

9. An advance to the net should always follow _____

   that has put your opponent on the _____.

10. Most opportunities to rush the net follow _____
    by your opponent.

11. The net position should be about _____

    behind the _____.

12. If you are caught in a poor position at the net, you should return

    with a volley _____ to reduce

    the _____.

13. When you have your opponent on the run, a good place to put the

    return is _____.

14. When playing from the baseline, you must return the ball _____

    _____ in the opponent's court.

15. What should you do if you realize that your opponent has a weak
    side and does not return ball well on that side?

    _____

16. When your opponent returns balls equally well from both sides, you

    should play the ball _____.

• •

Completion: The Doubles Game

1. In doubles, the team that controls the _____ will usually win.

2. The offense in doubles is built around the _____,

   _____, and _____.

3. The receiver's partner should position himself/herself:

   _____.

4. The server's partner should position himself/herself:

   _____.

5. How does the Double Bounce Rule affect the positions of the serving team? Why?

6. Which team has an advantage at the beginning of each point? Why?

7. The appropriate net position in doubles is _____.

8. When serving in doubles, where should the server stand?

   _____

9. In doubles, generally the serve should be placed _____

   to the receiver's _____.

10. If the partner of the server is standing up close to the non-volley zone, where should the receiver return the serve? Why?

11. For a deep serve in the outside corner of the even court, a

    _____ return is good.

12. The basic strategy in doubles play is for both partners to

    _____.

13. When a lob is made over the head of one player, what action should

    take place? _____

14. When the ball is hit down the middle of the court, which partner

    should return the ball? _____

15. If the opponent at the net continually drifts toward the center to poach, where should you return the ball?

    _____

• •

GAME OF PICKLE-BALL

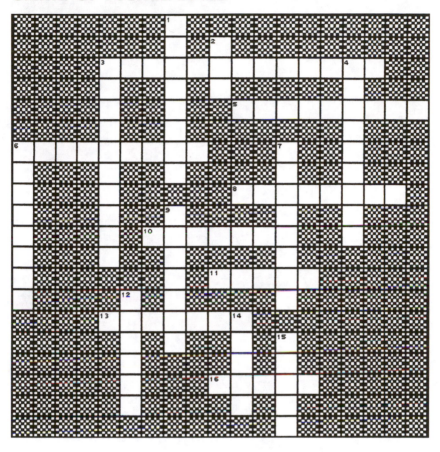

ACROSS CLUES
3. Presence at the net is a ____ advantage
5. In doubles the ____ team has one player up and one player back
6. Vary the pace and ____ of service
8. The ____ player should hit ball between two players.
10. Hard hit drive ____ net players will often result in a winner.
11. Distance from net is determined by ____ of opponent's serve
13. Serve returns should be deep to forehand or backhand ____
16. Baseline strategy lets the opponent make the ____

DOWN CLUES
1. Usually opponent's weakest return side
2. In doubles the ____ is the major defensive stroke
3. Major strategy in doubles is to take ____ of the net
4. Player can gain a distinct ____ when playing at the net
6. One player moving over to cut off ball usually played by partner
7. Mixed doubles has the player with ____ forehand in the middle
9. In doubles the ____ team must remain in backcourt until ball bounces
12. Receiver must allow ball to ____ before returning it
14. Rush net after a ____ return by opponent
15. Opponent likes to play back, so give him/her ____ balls to return

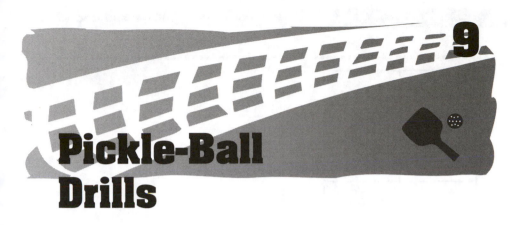

Pickle-Ball Drills

HAND-EYE COORDINATION DRILL

The key to Pickle-Ball is the ability to hit the ball with the paddle in a controlled manner. This involves perception, timing, and correct movement of the paddle. A simple but effective hand-eye coordination drill gives the student an opportunity to practice these skills individually by hitting the ball into the air. Proficiency is achieved when the student can hit 10 to 15 consecutive balls without moving more than two or three steps.

1. Find a place on the floor with room to swing the paddle freely.
2. Drop the ball, then swing the paddle with an underhand stroke at the ball.
3. Make contact with the ball, holding the arm relatively straight and the paddle head parallel to the floor.
4. After achieving reasonable control with the forehand, attempt the same drill with the backhand grip.
5. Alternate forehand and backhand strokes, being sure to modify the grip each time.

Also stroke the ball to the floor with the forehand grip to get used to how the ball will rebound from the floor.

COURT COVERAGE DRILL

Players must be able to move efficiently about the court and also to know where they are on the court at all times. This drill will help develop kinesthetic senses. It uses the lines of the badminton court for reference points (see Figure 9.1).

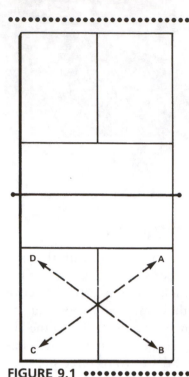

Court Coverage Drill.

FIGURE 9.1 •••

The starting point (X) is on the center service line approximately 12 feet from the net. Run to the intersection of the short service line and the right singles sideline boundary (A), do an underhand stroking motion, and return to the starting point (X). Next, slide quickly to the intersection of the doubles back service line and the right singles side boundary (B); do a drive stroking motion, and return to the starting point (X). Move to the intersection of the doubles back service line and the left singles side boundary (C); do a drive motion, and return to the starting point (X). Run to the intersection of the short service line and the left singles side boundary line (D); do an underhand stroking motion. Return to the starting point (X), and begin the drill again. This drill will be done for 30 seconds at maximum speed. Students must carry the paddle with the head held up at waist height at all times.

〰⊕ FIGURE 8 DRILL

All four doubles players are involved in this drill. A drives the ball down the sideline to B, who drives crosscourt deep to C. C drives down the sideline to D, who drives crosscourt deep to A. A begins the figure-8 path of the ball again. The ball should be kept deep in the corners of the court. A should be hitting fore-hand drives down the line, B hitting backhand crosscourts, C backhand drives down the line, and D hitting forehand cross-court drives (see Figure 9.2a).

Rotate players every 3 minutes so players practice all four locations. Volleys can also be practiced in this manner by mov-ing players up to just behind the non-volley zone (see Figure 9.2b).

⊜ DRIVE-AND-VOLLEY DRILL

A stands just behind the non-volley zone to volley the ball to B, who drives the ball to A. C and D do the same on the other side of the court. Change positions after about 4 minutes (see Figure 9.3).

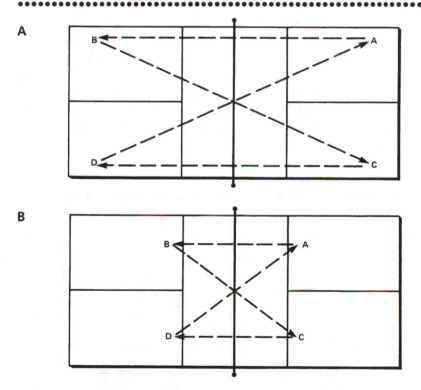

Figure 8 Drill.

FIGURE 9.2 ●●●

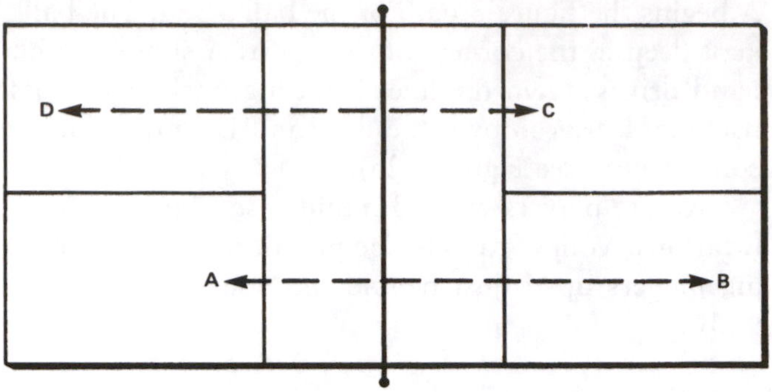

Drive-and-Volley Drill.

FIGURE 9.3

≈◉ SKILL DRILLS

Skill Drill #1: A Variety of Shots and Movements

Practice a variety of shots and movement. (1) Player A serves high to B who (2) returns the ball straight down the sideline. (3) Player A returns the drive with a drop shot straight over the net. (4) Player B returns the drop with a crosscourt lob deep in the court. Player A returns the lob with a drive down the sideline. Player B returns the drive with a drop shot straight over the net. Player A returns the drop with a crosscourt lob, starting the drill again (see Figure 9.4).

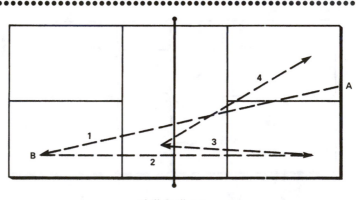

Skill Drill #1.

FIGURE 9.4

Skill Drill #2: Four Corners Singles Practice

This is a four-corner singles drill to practice down-the-line and crosscourt shots (see Figure 9.5).

    a. A hits down-the-line to B.

    b. B hits a crosscourt.

    c. A returns down-the-line.

    d. B hits another crosscourt.

    e. Reverse directions.

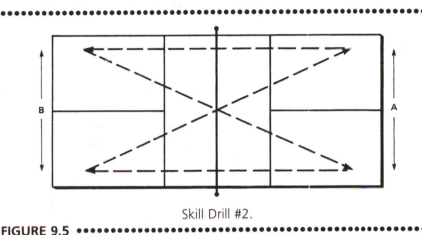

Skill Drill #2.

FIGURE 9.5

Skill Drill #3: Beginning Doubles Practice

A and B begin side by side, and C and D begin side by side in midcourt. B hits the ball midcourt to C. C return drops the ball in front of A. A crosscourt drops the ball in front of D. D lobs the ball back to B and the drill begins again. Players should keep a ball in hand to keep play continuous. Rotate players after a few minutes (see Figure 9.6).

Skill Drill #4: Player Reflexes

Players in this drill work on reflexes. Six players are on the court.

    a. A works for 2 minutes non-stop on volley and smashes (see Figure 9.7).

    b. B and C have balls. D and E route balls back to F, who gives them to B and C.

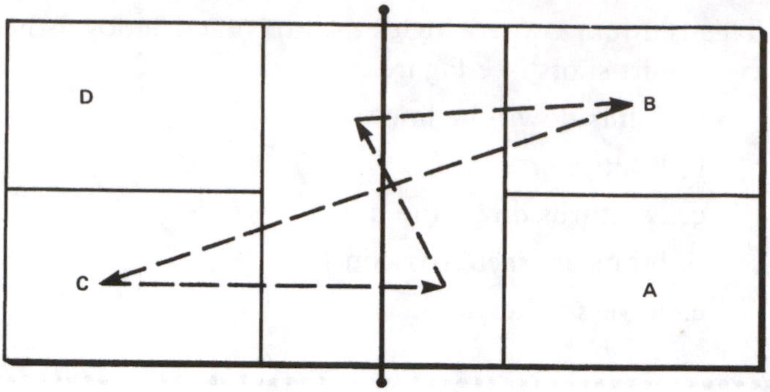

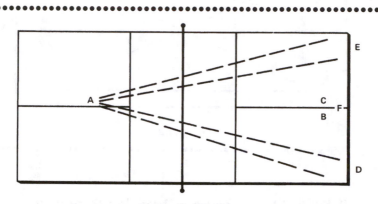

Beginning Doubles Practice.

FIGURE 9.6

Player Reflexes.

FIGURE 9.7

c. B, then C, hit balls to A, either to the sides or over him/her for a smash.

d. A must never stop hitting the ball. He/she hits all balls to the outside of B and C.

e. Rotate players after 2 minutes.

Skill Drill #5: Singles when Opponent is at Net

This gives the player specific practice in returning balls when opponent is at the net.

a. O at the net feeds playable balls to X.

b. X practices hitting to A or D area. These are difficult shots to make.

c. O does *not* try to return ball but just holds out paddle to the side to which the ball comes to see if it is reachable.

d. Player tries a high defensive lob, making certain the lob is deep into the court to one side or the other.

Have each player take six balls, then rotate players. When all have hit forehands, repeat the drill using the other side of the court for the backhand drill (see Figure 9.8).

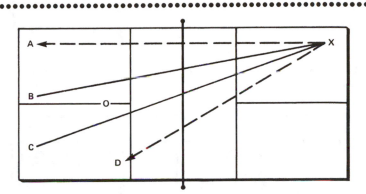

Singles Return when Opponent is at Net.

FIGURE 9.8 ●● ●●

Skill Drill #6: Alternating Drop and Lob

This is good for conditioning and learning to hit on the move. The non-volley zone must be observed.

Let the ball bounce. Player A will only hit drop shots to either side of the court. Player B will alternate hitting a drop followed by a lob. Example: B lobs deep — A overhand drops — B redrops — A redrops — B lobs (see Figure 9.9).

Skill Drill #7: Short Games

This game is played in the non-volley zone. The initial serve to put the ball in play is a drop shot from behind the non-volley zone. Score exactly like singles; any shot that goes beyond the non-volley zone is out (see Figure 9.10).

Skill Drill #8: Four Ball Attack

This drill gives practice in four basic shots. A has four balls. The first hit is a short drive to B's forehand. B returns the ball down the line. A next hits to B's forehand as B moves up to volley. A

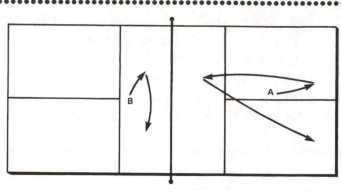

Alternating Drop and Lob.

FIGURE 9.9

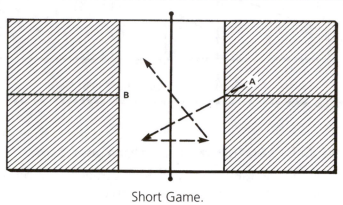

Short Game.

FIGURE 9.10

hits the third shot to B's backhand, which B volleys. A then hits the fourth ball — a midcourt lob for B moves back and hits with an overhead. Repeat with the backhand side (see Figure 9.11).

SUGGESTIONS FOR LARGE CLASSES WITH FEW COURTS

Double-Singles

A and B are playing against C and D. A will start against C. Both will take their respective serve turns. When the ball comes back to A, B will come in and play, adding any points gained to A's score. When the serve goes over to C, D will come in and

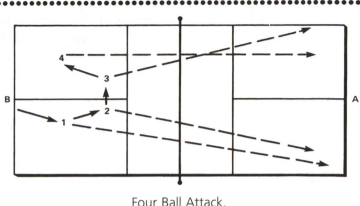

Four Ball Attack.

FIGURE 9.11

serve, adding any points to C's score. Keep switching until a game is played — 11 points with a 2-point lead.

Double-Doubles

A, B, C, and D are playing E, F, G, and H. A and B begin on the court against C and D. Both teams will take their respective terms of service. When the ball comes back to A and B for service, C and D will take the court and add any points gained to A and B's score. When the ball goes back to E and F, G and H will take the court and serve, adding points gained to E and F's score. Keep switching until a game is played — 11 points with a 2-point lead.

Scoring on Every Serve

With large classes and few courts, the side-out rule can be modified so a point is scored on every serve. This allows for a faster game with more people participating within a class period. One player serves for a total of five serves, then the opponent serves for five serves until one player scores 10 points (like table tennis).

Magic 10*

1. Students are divided into equal groups according to the number of courts available. Example: 4 courts, 32 students, will put 8 students on each court.

---

*Game devised by Jane Hooker, Memphis State University.

2. Two players, A and B, begin play using the no-side-out rule. Player A scores the point, remains on the court, and continues to serve. C, the next player in line, comes to challenge A and so on. Situation: A scores 2 points and then makes a fault, leaves the court but keeps the 2 points scored and goes to the end of the line. When it is his/her turn to return to the court, he/she keeps the 2 points and adds points until reaching 10 points. When a player reaches 10 points he/she moves up to the next court and begins a new game.

3. The object is to move to all four courts as quickly as possible.

Team Pickle-Ball*

Team Pickle-Ball was designed to allow physical education teachers to create maximum playing opportunities for students when court space is limited. A traditional volleyball court (30' x 60') is used for Team Pickle-Ball, with the net lowered to tennis height. Four to six players constitute a team.

In Team Pickle-Ball the 10-foot volleyball spiking line is used to establish the non-volley zone. The ball is served from the center of the court, at a spot 6 feet inside the back boundary line by the center back player when playing with five- or six-player teams, or by the right back player when playing with four-player teams.

Any player on the receiving team may play the served ball. The service, however, must bounce and clear the non-volley zone, anywhere in the backcourt. The serving team must also let the return of serve bounce, to observe the Double Bounce Rule. After these initial two plays, volleys are allowed, provided that players contact the ball from behind the non-volley zone and do not follow through into the non-volley zone.

Each team gets one hit to return the ball over the net. Points are scored only by the serving team. (You may play Score on Every Serve to speed the game along.) Receivers rotate as in volleyball after side-outs.

Hitting your own teammate with a return is a fault. In Team Pickle-Ball front-row players must learn to duck.

The first team to reach 11 points and is 2 points ahead wins the game. Two of three games constitutes a match.

---

*Game devised by Ricky Parris, Abilene Independent School District.

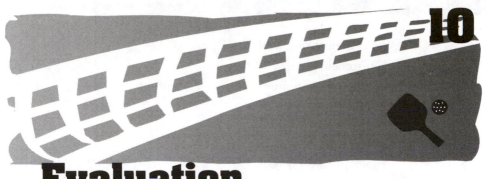

Evaluation

tudents want feedback on how they are progressing in developing their skills and knowledge in Pickle-Ball. Objective evidence of success motivates players to continue to strive for improvement with continued practice. Appropriate skill and knowledge tests will accurately assess a player's Pickle-Ball ability.

Evaluation should not be done just at the conclusion of the activity. It should be continuous, related to course objectives, and consist of activity-related skills.

KNOWLEDGE TESTS

Written examinations should evaluate the student's knowledge of material covered in class. Two or three short tests on specific areas covered during the course are preferred over a comprehensive final. For example, a test on the rules of Pickle-Ball could be given before students begin to play the game. This would allow the teacher to clear up any misunderstandings concerning scoring, odd and even courts, the Double-Bounce Rule, and so on. Later, students could be tested on terms, history, and strategy.

SKILL TESTS

Although skill testing takes time away from actual play, it is a valuable means of determining skill level. Tests should be administered during the course so the student can see how he or she is progressing toward established norms for the course.

The following battery of Pickle-Ball skills tests is being developed, and norms established for semester-length university courses.

I. Volley Against the Wall (see Figure 10.1)

1. Equipment needed:
   A. 16 balls minimum (4 per test station)
   B. Score sheets
   C. Pencils
   D. Stopwatch
   E. Small box for balls

2. Description of test:

   The player taking the test starts behind the restraining line with a paddle and *one* ball. The remaining three balls are placed in a box on the edge of the restraining line. If the player loses control of the ball, he/she must run to box to pick up the next ball. It cannot be handed to him/her. On the command "go," the ball is *volleyed* against the wall above the net line, and the player continues to *volley* the ball against the wall for *30 seconds. Balls hitting on or above the net line are counted.* If the restraining line is crossed, the hit is not counted, but the ball is still in play. Rotate all students before starting second and third trials.

   The test should be administered in groups of four students: #1 taking the test; #2 counting legal hits; #3 counting foot faults on legal hits to be subtracted from legal hits; #4 retrieving balls and placing them back in the box for his/her group.

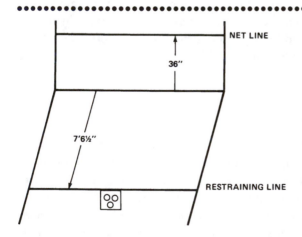

NET LINE

36"

7'6½"

RESTRAINING LINE

Volley against wall.

FIGURE 10.1

3. Scoring:

The score is the *average* of the three trials; drop any fractions. *Do not round up.*

II. Drive Against the Wall (see Figure 10.2).

1. Equipment needed:

A. 16 balls minimum (4 per test station)

B. Score sheets

C. Pencils

D. Stopwatch

E. Small box for balls

2. Description of test:

The player taking the test starts behind the restraining line with a paddle and *one* ball. The remaining three balls are placed in a box on the edge of the restraining line. If the player loses control of the ball, he/she must run to box to pick up the next ball. It cannot be handed to him/her. On the command "go," the ball is driven against the wall above the net line, and the player continues to drive the ball after it has bounced on the floor, for *30 seconds.* The *ball must hit the floor* before the player returns it to the wall. *Balls hitting on or above the net line are counted.* If the restraining line is crossed, the hit is not counted but the ball is still in play. Balls that have bounced more than once may be played. Rotate all students before starting second and third trials.

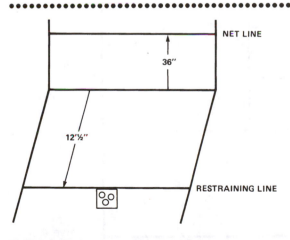

NET LINE

36"

12'½"

RESTRAINING LINE

Drive against wall.

FIGURE 10.2

The test should be administered in groups of four students: #1 taking the test; #2 counting legal hits; #3 counting foot faults on legal hits to be subtracted from legal hits; #4 retrieving balls and placing them back in the box for his/her group.

3. Scoring:

The score is the *average* of the three trials; drop fractions. *Do not round up.*

III. Serve Test (see Figure 10.3).

1. Equipment needed:

A. 16 balls

B. Score sheets

C. Pencils

D. Floor tape

E. Small box for balls

2. Description of test:

No practice serves shall be taken before actually beginning the test. All 15 serves shall be taken from the right-hand court, and be a *legal* serve. A ball touching the

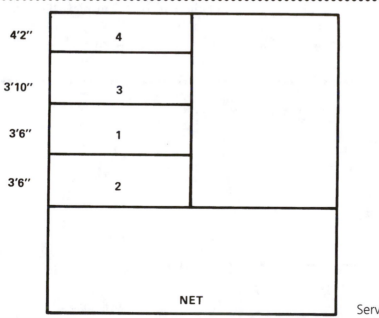

Serve test.

FIGURE 10.3

net and landing in the correct service court shall be re-served. A ball landing on a line shall receive the higher value.

3. Scoring:

The score shall be the total points accumulated on the 15 serves. (When a regulation badminton court is used, the 3-point area would be 4'8", not 3'10".)

The performance standards in Tables 10.1, 10.2, and 10.3 have been established with students from the Pickle-Ball classes at Abilene Christian University. Performance standards should be developed for each student population using these tests.

TABLE 10.1 ••
Performance Standards for Volley Test.

	SCORES	
Performance	Men	Women
Excellent	39–47+	28–36+
Good	33–38	20–27
Average	27–32	14–19
Fair	21–26	8–13
Poor...	0–20	0–7

••

TABLE 10.2 ••
Performance Standards for Drive Test.

	SCORES	
Performance	Men	Women
Excellent	26–30+	20–26+
Good	23–25	17–19
Average	20–22	13–16
Fair	17–19	10–12
Poor...	0–16	0–9

••

TABLE 10.3 ••
Performance Standards for Serve Test.

| | SCORES | |
Performance	Men	Women
Excellent	52–57+	48–53+
Good	47–51	42–47
Average	41–46	34–41
Fair	34–40	27–33
Poor..	0–33	0–26

Skill Test Recording Sheet

Name _____

Time _____ Teacher _____

I. Volley against wall:

        1._____   2._____   3._____

    Faults   ____   ____   ____   Grade

    Total   ____   ____   ____   Average _____   _____
                                                    (do not round up)

II Serving:

1	6	11
2	7	12
3	8	13
4	9	14
5	10	15

                                        Total_____   _____

III. Drive against wall:

        1._____   2._____   3._____

    Faults   ____   ____   ____   Grade

    Total   ____   ____   ____   Average _____   _____
                                                    (do not round up)

                                             Skills Test Grade _____

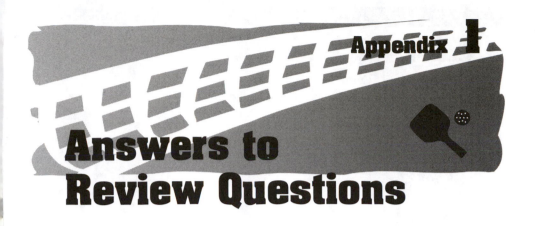

Answers to Review Questions

Chapter 1

1. where you want it
   tempo of the game
   the ball in play
2. badminton doubles court
3. 1965, Washington
4. a tree in the corner of the court would not obstruct the delivery
5. the Pritchard's dog, which ran off with the balls
6. an overpowering offensive weapon
7. net player's advantage
8. United States Pickle-Ball Association

Chapter 2

1. independent
2. sport
3. injuries
4. Anaerobic
5. aerobic
6. cardiorespiratory and muscular
7. Muscular strength
8. quadriceps and calf
9. obesity
10. muscle

Chapter 3

    1. 8 in., 15½ in.
    2. smooth, sandpaper, holes, glued granules
    3. 3 in.
    4. 20' x 44'
    5. 36 in./34 in.
    6. 7
    7. 3 to 5 ft.

Chapter 4

1. F	6. T
2. F	7. T
3. T	8. F
4. F	9. T
5. F	10. F

Chapter 5

1. F	7. F	13. T
2. T	8. F	14. F
3. F	9. T	15. F
4. F	10. T	16. T
5. T	11. T	17. T
6. T	12. F	18. T

Chapter 6

    1. Not showing up at all
    2. When point has finished
    3. Before any points are played
    4. a. Make sure receiver is ready
       b. Call out the score of the game
    5. Server's
    6. a. Let it go on past you
       b. Block it into the net after the bounce
    7. Return it over the net
    8. it is clearly out
    9. a. Wait until the point is over
       b. Politely say "thank you" or "ball, please."
  10. a. Wait until point is over
       b. Toss softly and accurately to nearest player
  11. Stop immediately and play a let

Chapter 7

1. F	5. F	9. T	13. F	17. T
2. T	6. F	10. T	14. T	18. F
3. F	7. T	11. F	15. F	19. F
4. F	8. F	12. F	16. F	20. T

Crossword Puzzle Answers: Pickle-Ball Terms

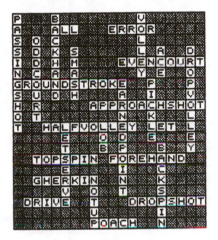

Chapter 8

Singles Game

1. near the center line
2. a couple of feet from the center line
3. a. deep to the far corners
   b. down the middle close to the center line
   c. directly at the receiver
4. a. Vary the pace
   b. Vary the placement
5. Held about shoulder high in front of the body
6. the speed of the opponent's serve
7. deep to corners
8. a weak return
9. a forcing shot, defensive
10. short shots
11. 2 feet, non-volley zone
12. deep down middle, angle of return
13. in the area of the court your opponent just left
14. deep

15. Hit the ball to that side
16. down the middle of the court.

Doubles Game
1. net
2. serve, volley, smash
3. at the net
4. back on baseline
5. Must let it bounce on first return, partner must be back
6. The receiving — already one partner at net
7. 2 feet behind non-volley zone and about 3 feet inside the sideline
8. halfway between center line and sideline, or slightly more to sideline.
9. deep, backhand
10. To partner at net, must let it bounce
11. down-the-line
12. gain the net
13. Both should retreat to baseline
14. Forehand player
15. Down the sideline

Crossword Puzzle Answers: Game of Pickle-Ball

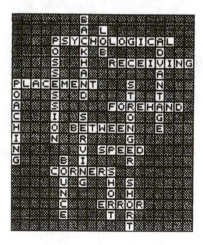

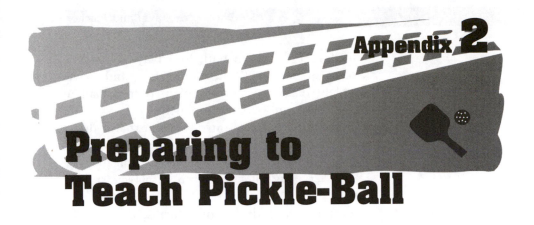

Preparing to Teach Pickle-Ball

Most teachers believe students should learn to execute skills in a setting similar to the game situation and play games or participate in game-like drills as soon as they develop the basic skills. Singles games should be played early in the unit if possible, for a player develops self-reliance and is forced to move efficiently on the court to play shots that the doubles partner would take. Throughout the unit each student should receive as much individual attention as possible from the teacher. The instructor should stress positive actions ("do this" instead of the negative "don't do that"). Students should be encouraged to analyze their own mistakes when they fail to hit the ball correctly.

PICKLE-BALL SKILLS VIDEO

A 15-minute videotape showing and explaining the basic skills has been developed. Skills included are the forehand and backhand drives, drive and lob serves, volley and drop volley, drop shot, smash, half-volley, and lob. Singles and doubles play are demonstrated. Three skills tests are shown and explained. This tape is available from Pickle-Ball, Inc.

OUTLINE FOR SEMESTER CLASS

Three Days a Week

DAY 1   Class orientation; explanation of the game of Pickle-Ball.

DAY 2   Explain parts of paddle, grips. Hand-eye coordination drill. Introduce volley and explain non-volley zone. Volley drills with partner — at net and Figure 8 pattern with four players. Practice volley off the wall. Introduce forehand drive. Explain ready position. Explain putting ball in play. Drive ball over net to partner.

DAY 3   Review volley drills. Introduce backhand drive, and do various drills for drive. Introduce drive serve and service rules. Explain Double Bounce Rule. Serve and play ball with all players staying in back court.

DAY 4   Court coverage drill. Volley drills, drive drills, drive serve practice. Drive and volley drill with partner. Serve and play point out, singles.

DAY 5   Court coverage drill. Review volley. Explain approach shot. Explain singles scoring. Play Double-Singles: two players keep their singles score together against other two singles partners.

DAY 6   Court coverage drill. Review drives and volley drills. Practice approach shot. Introduce lob serve. Play double-singles.

DAY 7   Court coverage drill. Introduce two types of lob and the smash. Play double-singles.

DAY 8   Go over Pickle-Ball etiquette. Explain half-volley. Play double-singles.

DAY 9   Court coverage drill. Introduce drop shot and drop volley. Practice lob and smash. Play double-singles.

DAY 10   Discuss singles strategy for service and return of service. Begin singles ladder challenge tournament.

DAY 11   Skill Drill #1. Discuss singles strategy of net play. Continue ladder tournament.

DAY 12   Discuss baseline strategy for singles. Continue ladder tournament.

DAY 13   Skill Drill #2. Continue ladder tournament.

DAY 14   Explain doubles scoring and position of partners on serve and receive of serve. Play doubles.

DAY 15   Skill Drill #3. Disucss strategy for serve and receive of serve. Play doubles.

DAY 16   Written test over skills, rules, and etiquette.

DAY 17   Discuss doubles net play strategy. Play doubles.

DAY 18   Discuss baseline play in doubles strategy. Play doubles.

DAY 19	Skill Drill #4. Play doubles.
DAY 20	Explain skills tests and practice them.
DAY 21–23	Begin doubles round robin tournament, 11 points, 2-point lead.
DAY 24	Skill Drill #5. Play singles.
DAY 25	Play singles.
DAY 26	Written test over singles and doubles strategy.
DAY 27	Practice volley and drive test. Play doubles.
DAY 28–29	Play singles.
DAY 30	Practice volley and drive test. Play doubles.
DAY 31–32	Play singles.
DAY 33	Practice volley and drive test. Play doubles.
DAY 34–35	Ladder singles tournament, two ladders, 7-point game.
DAY 36	Practice volley and drive test. Play doubles.
DAY 37–38	Continue ladder singles tournament.
DAY 39	Practice volley and drive test. Play doubles.
DAY 40–41	Continue singles ladder tournament.
DAY 42	Skill test on volley and drive.
DAY 43	Skill test on serve.
DAY 44	Written test over history and language of Pickle-Ball.

Two Days A Week

DAY 1	Class orientation, explanation of the game of Pickle-Ball.
DAY 2	Explain parts of the paddle, grips. Hand-eye coordination drill. Introduce volley and explain non-volley zone. Volley drills with partner, both at net, figure-8 pattern with four players at net. Practice volley off the wall. Introduce forehand drive. Explain ready position. Explain putting the ball in play. Drive ball over net to partner. Court coverage drill.
DAY 3	Review volley and forehand drive. Introduce backhand drive, and use various drills. Introduce drive serve and serve rules. Explain Double Bounce Rule. Serve and play out point, all stay back.
DAY 4	Court coverage drill. Review volley. Serve and play out point. Explain approach shot. Explain singles scoring. Play double-singles.

DAY 5	Review drives, volley, drive serve, and approach. Introduce lob serve. Play double-singles.
DAY 6	Court coverage drill. Introduce the lob, defensive and offensive. Introduce smash. Explain half-volley. Go over Pickle-Ball etiquette. Play double-singles.
DAY 7	Court coverage drill. Introduce drop shot and drop volley. Review lob and smash. Play double-singles.
DAY 8	Discuss singles strategy of service and return of service. Begin singles ladder tournament.
DAY 9	Skill Drill #1. Discuss singles strategy of net play. Continue singles ladder tournament.
DAY 10	Skill Drill #2. Discuss singles strategy of baseline play. Continue singles ladder tournament.
DAY 11	Explain doubles scoring and positions. Play doubles.
DAY 12	Skill Drill #3. Discuss doubles strategy of serve and receive. Play doubles.
DAY 13	Test over skills rules and etiquette. Play after test.
DAY 14	Discuss doubles strategy of net play and baseline play. Play doubles.
DAY 15	Explain skills tests and practice them.
DAY 16	Skill Drill #4. Doubles round robin tournament.
DAY 17–18	Doubles round robin tournament.
DAY 19	Test over singles and doubles strategy. Play singles after test.
DAY 20	Skill Drill #5. Play singles.
DAY 21	Play singles.
DAY 22	Practice volley and drive skill tests. Play singles.
DAY 23	Ladder singles tournament.
DAY 24	Practice volley and drive skills tests. Continue ladder singles tournament.
DAY 25	Singles ladder tournament.
DAY 26	Practice volley and drive skills tests. Continue ladder singles tournament.
DAY 27	Practice serve skills test. Continue ladder singles tournament.
DAY 28	Take all skills tests.
DAY 29	Written test over history and language of Pickle-Ball. Finish any skills tests not completed.

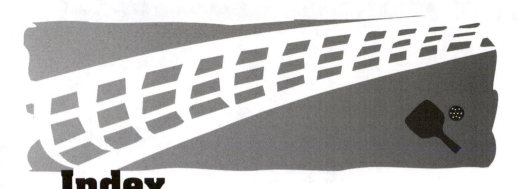

Index